Think, Act, Love,
Lose Weight

The 10 Secrets To
Forever Weight Loss

Shane Jeremy James

Think, Act, Love, Lose, Weight

Resource www.thinkactloveloseweight.com

ISBN-13:

978-0615474410 (Shane Jeremy James)

Empowering Nations International, Inc.

Design by Justin Oefelein of SPX Multimedia
Exercise Illustrations by Justin Oefelein

Disclaimer and legal information

The advice in this book may not be suitable for everyone. Information in this book regarding nutritional supplements, specific foods and exercise programs are not intended to replace appropriate necessary medical care. Require a physician before starting any exercise program. If you have certain medical symptoms, consult your physician. The author designed the information to present his beliefs about the subject matter. The reader should take all necessary steps to investigate all aspects of any decision before committing him or herself. The purchaser of this publication assumes full responsibility for the use of these materials and information. The publisher and author assume no liability whatsoever on behalf of any reader of this material.

Table of Contents

Dedication

To my Grandma and Grandpa, who have always believed in me and stuck by my side. Thank you for all the years of support. We have had so many good times, and have so many great memories. There is nothing I have appreciated more in this world than our time together. This book is dedicated to you.

Dedication

To my best friend and business partner, Jennifer, thank you for all your support in helping make all my dreams come true. I have enjoyed our journey together, and look forward to many more years to come. You are a living example of unconditional love and support, and the smartest businesswoman I know. You are an inspiration in this world. Thank you.

To my Mom, who has always been there by my side, through the good times and the bad times. I would not be the person I am today if you had not supported me when I really needed it. I could not ask for a better mom.

To my Dad, whom I always knew I could turn to when I needed to. Thanks for being there for me, being a part of my life, and helping with this book launch. I am excited for many more great years to come.

To my Grandma and Grandpa James, who never got a chance to see this book launched. However, I do know you are watching from above. I will always love you and miss you with all my heart.

To my brother, who is the most loyal person that I know. There is nothing that could ever come between us. Thanks for being someone I can always count on, no matter what happens in our lives. You have always had my back, and I will always have yours. There is nothing more rewarding than knowing I have a brother I can count no matter what.

To my PR agent, Imal Wagner, by far the best PR agent in the business. Thanks for taking the time with me, teaching me so much, believing in me. You really walk your talk, and want your clients to succeed at an extraordinary level. You're a great friend, and I look forward to many more business endeavors together.

To my auntie Ellen, thank you for taking the time to step up and help me with the book when I really needed it. This book came to completion because of your help. I appreciate it so much.

To Lil, my main editor of the book, who got the job done in a rush with no complaints. It has been such a pleasure to work with you. I look forward to many more years of business success and great friendship.

Thank you to my best friend, Kelly Bangert, who wrote the foreword for the book. Not only do you understand how to make millions of dollars, more importantly, you are a great friend and family man. It was like we were brothers the first time we met. I am happy to have you in my life.

Justin, who did the design of the book and all my CD programs, your work is great and the speed with which you get things done is hard to find. I look forward to many more years of friendship and business success together.

I would like to thank one of mentors, John Volken. You always give me the time to come and see you and all the business advice I need. It's a privilege to be a part of your life.

I would like to thank you, the reader, for opening up your mind to new possibilities. Whatever you believe, you really can achieve. I am a walking example.

Forward

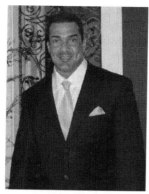

By Kelly Bangert

Shane Jeremy James understands how to help people lose weight. He knows the most important part of losing weight is to first change your thinking. He understands why fad diets don't work, and would never create one. The truth is, if I could describe my friend Shane, I would say he is by far one of the most motivated people I have ever met in my life. He will do whatever it takes to help you get lasting results.

When I first met Shane, we connected instantly, and to this day are like brothers. I could not think of anybody better for you to learn from to achieve all your weight and life goals. I believe Shane rose so fast in the motivational speaking area because of one thing, and that's his ability to connect with people. He really cares about people and their success. I think that's why he has been dubbed "the people's guru". He will do whatever it takes, for as long as it takes to help you achieve your goals.

He understands human behavior and human psychology better than most people I know. This really separates him from any other weight loss expert. Shane has also walked in your shoes; he has had the struggles you have had with your weight issues, and he has found ways to lose the weight and keep it off forever. Shane has never yo-yo dieted. He lost the weight and never gained it back; and that's when he created the program you are presented with in this book. There is great power in that, and you should understand that if you model what Shane has done, you can get the exact same results. This book is written by somebody who truly understands what it takes to lose the weight, but more importantly, lose the weight forever.

One of the things I appreciate about this book is that Shane doesn't preach at you from a high level; he speaks to you and teaches you like a trusted friend, who just happens to be extremely motivated, and has learned and discovered principles that most people don't know. He brings these principles to you in a way that is easy to learn and understand. Shane goes in-depth into the aspects of changing your psychology and mindset, but he doesn't stop there. He then teaches you everything you need to know about nutrition, and gives you a full exercise program you can do at home. To me, this is a well-rounded weight loss book. Before I wrote this foreword, I looked at many other weight loss books on the market, and most were missing certain aspects to really help people change their weight and keep it off forever. Some would talk about the mind, but had nothing to say about nutrition; others would talk about nutrition, but not about the mind. Others would just talk about exercise, but not about the other two. This is why most of these other programs just give people false hope. You will notice a common theme in this book. There are no exaggerated theories or sales pitches to gain your attention. All the information is true, sound advice to create lasting change in your weight.

Shane has not only become one of my best friends, but we have also done business together. In his business life, he understands more than anybody the importance of having a strong mind, confidence, passion, and a strong belief system. He brings those same traits from his highly successful business world into the weight loss world. You get a lot more in this book than just the principles of weight loss. This book has the potential to shape your whole life. Shane is an unbelievable teacher, mentor, and friend, and if you ever get a chance to meet him in person, you will understand what I mean.

Kelly grew up with a single mom and an older brother and sister, on welfare. They were very poor during his childhood, and received public assistance and food stamps for many years. He wore his brother's hand-me-down clothing, and did not experience new clothes until he was sixteen and had a job of his own. At the age of 21, Kelly became a police officer. He was struck by tragedy, injured in the line of duty, and medically retired from the police department. After that, Kelly started numerous businesses, and quickly made well over three million dollars. He is also one of the seven highest income earners in the direct sales industry - worldwide. Kelly made $3,408,500 in just nine months in the direct sales industry.

Introduction

As I stood in the bookstore, looking at all the different diet books, I counted over 100 books claiming to have the best solution. I am an expert in the weight loss industry and even I was getting confused. How must the average person feel? Overwhelmed, confused, and frustrated, I would imagine.

Every month a new guru comes out with a weight loss book, or a well-known guru repackages his message in a different way. And yet, according to the World Health Organization, one billion adults are overweight, and at least 300 million of them are clinically obese. If people keep gaining weight at the current rate, fat will be the norm by 2015, with 75 percent of U.S. adults overweight, and 41 percent of them obese. As you're reading this, every 18 minutes someone dies of diet-related health issues, and not only obese people, but also those who are "just" overweight. Diet-related diseases are the biggest killer in the United States today.

And the problem is not restricted to the U.S.; it is becoming a global epidemic. It even has a name: globesity. The majority of countries in the world have mass numbers of overweight and obese people.

When I pulled each and every one of those weight loss books off the shelf and skimmed through them, it was not hard to figure out why the mass majority of them do not work. Let's be honest. If they did work, the world's population would not be getting fatter and fatter, and we would not be dying at a rapid rate from this problem. A large portion of these diet books that I read through are just a cash grab making the gurus selling them millions of dollars, and giving people false hope in their moment of weakness.

We have all heard the saying, "If you keep doing the same things, you will keep getting the same results." That's what happens with most people trying to lose weight. They go from book to book, program to program, guru to guru, and never get lasting results.

My commitment to you is to show you the only way that you can lose the weight and keep it off forever. This challenge is designed so that you never again have to pick up another weight loss book, hope for another guru to come along with something new, or be manipulated by the clever marketing techniques in the weight loss industry that give you a false sense of hope.

Together, we are going to create a healthy nation. This will be the biggest movement that you will ever be involved in. Right now the world is ready for something completely different. You are about to be part of something that has never been done before. We are going to totally revolutionize the weight loss industry.

It is important to me that you realize that I have walked in your shoes. I am not one of those experts who is going to teach you how to lose weight and say I know how you feel when I have never been there.

In this book, you will learn the strategies that transformed me from being an extremely unhappy person, addicted to drugs, 65 pounds overweight, broke, with no place to live, and with no sense of direction, to a centered, in-shape, healthy individual who beat food and a drug addictions. Today, I not only have great relationships and the opportunity for unlimited success, but I am also being mentored by millionaires, becoming financially free, and appearing on TV. I have become a best-selling author, co-authoring books with the likes of Tony Robbins, Brian Tracy, and Dr. Wayne Dyer, while I live my dream of being a motivational speaker. Most importantly, I have the privilege of helping hundreds of thousands of people across the world live better lives.

I was just a small town boy who grew up in a town of 1000 people on the prairies in Canada, when I left with some really big dreams and moved to a city of over 2 million people. If I can overcome the struggles that I have overcome, each and every one of you has the ability to create whatever you want in this world. I am going to show you how. Even though this book is about weight loss, you will be able to apply the many strategies and techniques you will learn in all areas of your life. Each and every one of you has the power to transform your body and life, and to achieve your greatest dreams.

Have you noticed that most weight loss programs on the market promote their products with messages such as: eat fewer calories than you burn; exercise more; eat low carb, no carb, high protein, low protein? We saw the Atkins craze explode overnight and then disappear the next day. These diet fads have been coming and going for the last 50 years. For you to lose weight and keep it off forever you have to have a bigger vision than just to lose weight. You have to be part of something that will change the world. It has to be about more than just you; it has to become about helping create a healthy nation. People are only truly motivated when they have a greater vision, and a strong enough why.

If you and I can think it, we can create it; we can and we will create a healthy nation. The truth is, one person, one city, or one country cannot beat this weight epidemic alone. But together, we can create something much bigger, deeper, and more powerful than just the next diet book or weight loss fad.

Human behavior studies have proven that people are much more motivated to achieve something when they are competing in a challenge. That is why shows like The Biggest Loser are so successful. Most hit reality TV shows involve some kind of challenge, with a reward at the end. I finally got tired of everyone watching people on TV shows like The Biggest Loser get results and cheer the winners on, while the rest of the nation sits on the couch and gains weight. The only real winners are the ones on the shows.

In this challenge, you will learn the most important aspects of losing weight and keeping it off forever. The first steps may be familiar, but weight loss books on the market either do not teach them or do not go into enough depth. That's why most of these diet books and weight loss programs do not work. Sure, they can help you lose weight, but they don't help you keep it off forever. When you combine all these steps together, it is by far the most powerful way on the planet to lose weight.

My goal is not just to help you lose weight. My goal is to show you how to keep it off for the rest of your life. My promise to you now is, I will be your weight loss and health coach for the rest of your life. That's why they call me "the people's guru," because I care about one thing, and that is helping you add many healthy years to your life.

Here is the secret formula for long-term weight loss success. What makes this program truly unique is that I am one of the leading experts in personal achievement and one of the leading experts in the weight loss industry. When you combine the two together, personal achievement and weight loss, you get something that is extremely powerful —the missing link in the weight loss industry. Most of the gurus in the weight loss industry are just trained in one thing, weight loss. They are not experts in personal achievement, so a lot of the programs just do not work.

Step one
In-depth personal achievement

The only way to lose weight and keep it off forever is to learn how to change your behaviors. You have to change the way you think and act, and change the behaviors that you have been engaging in over and over again for years. This is by far the most important step. Exercising more and eating fewer calories does not work unless you first change the way you have been doing things. We all know that we have to exercise and eat healthy, so why can't we get ourselves to do it on a consistent basis? It's what's going on in our inner world that creates our outer world. In each chapter, we go in-depth and change thoughts, emotions, and behaviors that have been holding you back from success for years. This is the only way to lose weight and keep it off forever. I will give you lots of strategies that will help you in all areas of your life. When you're done with this book, you will be a completely different person.

Step two
Motivation through challenge

Motivation through challenge goes a long way. As human beings, from a young age we're motivated to compete. It has been proven that we have a far greater chance of succeeding at weight loss when we are part of some kind of challenge. A challenge will push you and those around you to a new level. Once I teach you how to create a strong enough why, and you combine that with a challenge, the chance of long-term success in your change initiative increases 100 percent.

Step three
Reach out and help someone

Select the person or people you will take the challenge with. This is an extremely important step that will keep you motivated to follow through. I disagree with the statement that in order to help others, you first must help yourself. When you reach out and help someone else take this challenge, you will be automatically helping yourself. You will gain motivation and strength, and have the ability to improve your own situation at the same time. Even if someone lives in a different city, reach out to them and take the challenge together. You can keep track of each other by Internet and phone.

Step four
Share the challenge

Being part of something that can change the world will give you a massive amount of motivation. You must understand that one person can make a huge difference. Everyone needs to feel a sense of belonging, and to feel that you can really make a difference in the world and help people. You are now part of something much bigger and more powerful than just losing weight or reading another diet book. You have the power to help change the world and many people's lives through competing and sharing in this challenge.

Step five
Personal achievement and exercise combined

Now to the exercise portion. This is what every weight loss book focuses on: You have to exercise more and change your diet. We have heard this over and over. But without the first four steps above, very few of these programs will ever give you long-term results. I have developed one of the most effective and efficient exercise programs on the planet for you to achieve your ideal, healthy weight. We all know we need to exercise, but the problem is committing to doing it day after day. I will teach you the secrets that will help you stay with it for the rest of your life, and give you long-term results. The main reason I want you to implement exercise for the rest of your life is not just to be lean, but to add many healthy years to your life, and enjoy a great quality of life as you get older.

Step six
Eat to live

This is the eating portion of the program. I'm going to teach you how to eat healthy. My goal is not to put you on a diet, because diets don't work. When I lost 65 pounds, I did not go on a diet. That's why I have been able to keep it off. I am going to show you how to integrate healthy eating into your lifestyle so it just becomes a part of your everyday routine. Most diets are not designed to become a part of your everyday routine for the rest of your life. And over time, many of these diets are likely to damage your health.

We are going to change negative patterns that you have likely been practicing for years and years, such as going from one diet to the next. First you lose the weight, then you gain it back, then you lose it, then you gain it back again. My goal in this food section is to show you how you can add many healthy years to your life, and increase your quality of life while reducing your waistband. This eating plan will even help you slow down the aging process. Now do I have your attention?

This program is more of a lifestyle program than it is a weight loss program. It is important for you to understand why you're engaged in a daily battle with excess weight. You're overweight because of your overall lifestyle, not just because you eat too much and don't exercise enough.

Welcome to our 90-day challenge!

1. Find at least one person to take this challenge with you. If you don't have a partner, you can still be part of the challenge, but I highly suggest that you have a partner. If you can get more than one partner, go for it! The more, the merrier.

2. Read at least one chapter per day; more if you would like.

3. Stand in front of the mirror naked.
   We're not doing this to make you feel bad about yourself. I just want you to start to be honest with yourself. Assess where you are right now, and realize that you are not a bad person because you are overweight. I want you to love yourself the way you are right now, and I want you to get excited about the changes that you are going to make. As you look in the mirror, realize that we all have different body structures. When you get to your ideal, healthy weight, most likely, you're not going to look like a celebrity or a supermodel. Get comfortable with yourself, and accept that no two people are the same.

   Look in the mirror and say, "I love myself."

4. Measure yourself, but don't focus on the scale. Studies have shown that your weight is not the most important concern; your waist circumference matters more. Just because every celebrity worries about his or her weight does not mean it's the right way to do things. Remember this pro-

gram is all about changing your thinking, and giving you completely new ways to do things. We're going to focus on measuring your waist, rather than measuring your weight. It is important for you to realize that, due to where your organs are, belly fat is the most dangerous. You will measure your waist every week. You can take one peek at the scale when you start, just to give you a baseline. Then, you will only check on day 15, day 30, day 45, day 60, day 75, and day 90. That's seven trips to the scale in three months. You don't need to be running to the scale daily to check your weight. It's not that important. And I am going to teach you how to build some muscle to burn more body fat. Muscle weighs more than fat. That's one more good reason not to focus on the scale.

5. Most of us are so conditioned to track our progress with a scale, we don't even realize that being a slave to it is not working. You need to track your overall health. How many healthy years are you going to add to your lifespan? Take your blood pressure to see where you really are in terms of overall health. Your normal blood pressure should be at an optimum level of 115/76. First, take your reading three times a day: once in the morning, once in the afternoon, and again in the evening. Taking the average of all three readings will give you an accurate measurement. Don't take your blood pressure for 30 minutes after you work out, when it will be higher. After the initial reading, you should check your blood pressure once per month to measure your progress. If your blood pressure is high, you may need to track it daily.

6. Start an exercise routine that works with your schedule. See exercise section.

7. Review the diet and eating sections, and go shopping. If you're taking the challenge with one or more partners, shop together.

8. Measure and weigh yourself.

9. Take a photo of yourself, so you can compare the before and after shots.

10. Sign a contract to yourself, and hang it where you can see it every day.

11. Get a journal or notebook, and journal daily.

12. Find a picture of the exact body you would like to have. Make sure the person in the picture has a similar body structure to yours. Put this picture in front of you every time you work out.

13. Put an elastic band around your wrist. To reinforce healthy eating habits, snap yourself with the elastic band when you are making bad food choices. Do this every day until the challenge is over. Use it when you need to after the challenge has ended.

14. Reward yourself with small rewards at the end of each week, but only if you have followed though.

The top three winners will receive a personal reward from Shane Jeremy James. See rules for what you need to do to qualify to win prizes.

First prize will be an all expense paid trip for you and one other person to a secret location for a weekend of relaxation and fun. Shane Jeremy James will be joining you, so you will continue to learn many new secrets on how to become more successful.

Why are personal rewards so important? Relying on self-discipline is not always enough. If you want to lose weight, you need a strong personal incentive. Why? Because a good incentive reminds you that you are doing something you want to do, not something you have to do. A good incentive helps you to stay on track when you encounter temptation. Ideally, find a totally selfish reason to reach your ideal, healthy weight, a concrete benefit to look forward to. And keep reminding yourself of it, every day.

Rules to win the challenge

- *Take before and after pictures.*

- *Write down your starting weight and measurements, and your ending weight and measurements.*

- *Take the challenge for 12 consecutive weeks.*

- *Write about how this experience has had an impact on your life.*

- *Send us your before and after pictures, and your starting and ending weight and measurements, along with your write-up on how this experience has changed your life, and we will select our winners.*

How to keep you and your challenge partner(s) motivated:

- *Shop together weekly for healthy groceries.*

- *Schedule a time each day to do the exercises together. If you can't be together, check in with your partner to make sure they do their exercise routine that day.*

- *Pay a dollar each time you miss a workout.*

Measure and weigh

Day 1 _____
Measure your waist circumference and total weight.

Day 5 _____
Measure your waist circumference.

Day 10 _____
Measure your waist circumference.

Day 15 _____
Total weight.

Day 20 _____
Measure your waist circumference.

Day 25 _____
Measure your waist circumference.

Day 30 _____
Total weight.

Day 35 _____
Measure your waist circumference.

Day 40 _____
Measure your waist circumference.

Day 45 _____
Total weight.

Day 50 _____
Measure your waist circumference.

Day 55 _____
Measure your waist circumference.

Day 60 _____
Measure your total weight.

Day 65 _____
Measure your waist circumference.

Day 70 _____
Measure your waist circumference.

Day 75 _____
Total weight.

Day 80 _____
Measure your waist circumference.

Day 85 _____
Measure your waist circumference.

Day 90 _____
Measure your waist circumference and total weight.

NOTES:

CHAPTER ONE
The Secret To Weight Loss Mastery

You have the power to transform your life

The secret to weight loss mastery is not a cookie-cutter approach that claims to work for everyone. What I have to offer you is an individualized approach that will work for you. This is a program for developing a lifelong commitment to weight loss and good health that will work, because it will be designed by, and for, you. You will become the master of your own destiny.

This book is about much more than just how to lose weight. It's about changing how you think, and achieving self-mastery – mentally, emotionally, and physically. Leonardo da Vinci, an artistic and scientific virtuoso, once said:

One can have no smaller or greater mastery than mastery of oneself.

With this understanding, Leonardo not only became one of the world's greatest painters, but also a musician, scientist, architect, engineer, geologist, botanist, and writer. You too have the power to paint the fresco of your own life.

What makes this book truly unique is that you can apply the principles and strategies I'm going to teach you not only to your weight loss goals, but to all your life goals. Thousands of my seminar participants and weight loss clients have written to me, saying, "You have not only helped me change my weight, you have helped me change my life."

You have the ability to direct your own thoughts and behaviors, and produce outstanding results. I will show you how to improve your health and add extra years to your life. But first, you must come to terms with the reality that your weight issues start in the mind. A healthy mind produces a healthy body.

If you have ever failed on a diet, this book is for you. Implement the strategies I will teach you, and you will:

- Lose weight and keep it off for a lifetime
- Control your cravings
- Stop your endless counting of calories, fats, and carbs
- Detoxify your body
- Slow down the aging process
- Increase your energy and motivation
- Create a new way of thinking in all areas of your life
- Gain complete control over yourself once and for all
- Elevate your quality of life

Self-mastery is easier than you may think. Most people have no idea the enormous capacity for change we possess when we focus all of our resources on mastering a single area of our lives. Scientific research shows that you do have the capacity to break old habits; change your beliefs and perceptions; master new skills; and become a totally new person. Read this book, and you will have all the resources you need at your disposal to master yourself, mentally, emotionally, and physically. I promise you that.

Never doubt the power of your mind

I'll never forget the day that I suddenly realized I had achieved everything that I had envisioned for myself. As I drove my BMW to one of my weight loss seminars, I was talking on my cell phone to a multi-millionaire who was offering me his assistance to help advance my career. I was healthy and fit; in place of that extra sixty-five pounds of unwanted fat protruding over my belt, I could feel my strong abs supporting me with every breath. I no longer needed a quick fix of empty calorie foods to boost my mood. And I was bursting with positive energy.

I drove past the bus stop where, a mere seven years before, I used to catch the bus every day. In those days, I was concerned about having enough money for bus fare or a McDonald's cheeseburger. I had no real direction, no focus, no sense of identity. The only escape I could find from the emptiness I felt was through food, drugs, or alcohol. Constantly substituting one addiction for another, I felt scared and alone.

But as I drove by in my BMW that day, I thought about what a huge difference seven years can make. And I realized that all of the challenges in my past had paved the way for the extraordinary way of life that I now enjoyed.

Making changes in beliefs and behaviors

We have all experienced changes that have lasted for only a day, a week, a month, or maybe even a year. But what we are after here is not a short-term fix; our goal is to create change that lasts a lifetime. We are not talking about just making a change in the way you eat, but a change in you as a person; we're talking about changing the way you think and behave to create a new and more powerful you.

You will stop thinking like a human garbage disposal who constantly overeats, and start thinking like a thin, fit person who makes healthy food and lifestyle choices. Imagine how good a healthy diet will make you feel. You can have that feeling for a lifetime. You will become a person who shapes your own life. You have the power. You have control over all of your choices. You are the painter of your life's masterpiece. So no more justifications, no more excuses; the time to change is now.

I learned to model people who had already made the changes I wanted to make. What did these successful people have in common? How did they think? What did they believe? How did their beliefs affect their behavior? What did they do differently to create lasting change? Learn to ask good questions. The quality of your questions will determine the quality of your results.

I can ask a person just five questions, and be able to identify the core problems and insecurities that hold them back from success. Then we work together to change those unsupportive beliefs, enabling them to shed their insecurities and their excess weight for the rest of their life.

Later, we will take a tour deep into the subterranean level of the mind, the unconscious, and explore how we can change our lives by changing our deeply rooted beliefs. But first, let's take a closer look at the core concepts and strategies that you will be using to guide yourself on this journey.

Raise your level of success

If you incorporate the strategies I teach into your life, you will raise your level of success from where you are now to heights you can now only imagine. You will bring the "impossible" into the realm of what's possible for you. The first step on that journey is to simply make a decision. Once you decide the level of success you want to reach, and define what that looks like for you, you will set in motion all the other wheels that will keep you rolling in the right direction.

The path to raising your level of success is no mysterious "magic bullet"; reinventing your life requires discipline and hard work. Like the samurai, who rose to become the elite warrior class of Japan, you must cultivate discipline. Master yourself mentally, emotionally, and physically, and you will automatically raise your level of success.

What is it going to take for you to create lasting changes in your life? What will truly light that fire within you that will cause you to take control of your mind, your emotions, and your body once and for all? If you are going to create the body, the success, and the life that you have always wanted, you can't be trying to build that success on a hope or a wish. Each goal must become a "have-to"; something you have to have. In chapter three, we will explore how to find your true source of inspiration. For now, let me just plant the seed in your mind that finding the right motivation is critical to your success.

To raise your level of success, anything you set your mind to must become a "have-to". You must be willing to do whatever it takes to succeed. The only difference between people who achieve their goals and those who don't is the willingness to do whatever it takes.

How do you know if you're moving in the right direction? If you're doing the same things over and over, and achieving total success in your life, keep doing those things! Most of us keep doing the same things we have always done, and expect different results. The excess weight will never come off if you keep doing the same things you have always done. To achieve different results, you need to change what you are doing and how you are doing it. Start doing things differently and you will be working toward success.

Every day, ask yourself what you are doing differently to raise your level of success. It could be something as simple as getting up an hour earlier in the morning to fit in a workout. If your goal is to create more love and affection in your life, maybe it's telling ten people you love them today. There are an infinite number of ways to raise your level of success. Become aware of the things that are not bringing you any closer to your goals, and do something different!

Let's start with thinking differently. A belief is simply a thought that you hold to be one hundred percent true. To change anything in your life, you must first change your limiting beliefs. Instead of supporting your success, these beliefs hold you back from achieving everything you desire. So start to question your beliefs, and adopt new ones that will serve you on your journey to success.

While we're on the subject of beliefs, let's talk about your belief in your own ability to succeed. Do you think that if you have a 99.9% belief in yourself, you can succeed? No! Just one-tenth of a percent of doubt can hold you back. Doubt is insidious; even the tiniest seed of doubt can prevent you from achieving your goals and aspirations. You must create a "without-a-doubt" mindset. Do not doubt yourself; there are enough other people in the world that will do that for you.

There will be no shortage of people on your journey who will tell you that your dream is unachievable. Some will scoff at your claim that you are not only going to lose the excess weight, but keep it off forever. They may say, "You've failed in the past. What makes you think you can succeed this time?" Or, "Why bother with another weight loss program when you've failed with all the others?" Do any of these dream-killing words sound familiar? Others may not douse your dreams outright; they just may not offer any encouragement.

Often, the reason other people do not support your dreams is that they do not believe that they themselves could do it. When you decide to make a change, when you stretch beyond your "comfort zone", you challenge their view of reality because they don't believe in their own ability to succeed. Even those who love us may get uncomfortable with any major changes we make in our lives. Don't buy into other people's limiting beliefs! You get to choose which beliefs to adopt; why not choose supportive ones?

Choose to believe in yourself with one hundred percent conviction. Don't let doubt fueled by past failures creep into your mind. You are learning to do things differently this time. And it all starts with changing the way you think.

Find a strategy that works

Once you have the right attitudes in place – you are disciplined, you are doing things differently, you believe in yourself without-a-doubt – are you ready to succeed? Not yet. Next you need to find the right strategy, the one that will work for you.

Japanese warriors used hundreds of sword fighting techniques. But what set the elite samurai apart were the distinctive techniques and unique sequences they developed that put them in a class of their own. For example, they developed the technique of drawing and slicing a sword in a single, fluid motion. Actually a precise series of steps, this allowed them to defeat their opponent quickly and decisively. If they failed to perform the sequence exactly right, they would not succeed with their strike.

Similarly, the highly customizable weight loss strategy I have developed for you is in that elite "samurai" class. How is it different from any other diet or weight loss program? The sequence of the steps is the key to achieving long-term results. Placed in a different order, the same steps will not work. You cannot build a house without the required foundation. You can't run a car on an empty gas tank. Foundation first. Gas first. Reshape your mind before you reshape your body.

Many weight loss programs fail to create long-term results because they are running on empty, and they don't address your total health – a healthy mind, body, and spirit. They often start with the advice to simply exercise more and eat less. But if you don't have a strong foundation to support your success, of course you will fail! If you don't adopt the mindset of success, and believe without-a-doubt that you can achieve your goals, you will not have the ability to make permanent healthier lifestyle choices.

The strategy I will help you design will change your unsupportive beliefs, keep you motivated, and ultimately, help you to maintain your new, healthy weight for a lifetime. Realize that when it comes to gaining control over your weight, you have not failed; the strategies you have been using have failed you. All those other misguided weight loss programs, diet books, and gurus have failed you. Provided you have the right tools to use in the right sequence, you will lose the excess weight – and keep it off forever.

One size does not fit all

When I was going to school, I was a "problem student". I wouldn't sit still; I didn't listen; I always seemed to be focused on something other than what was being taught. Why did teachers typically have such a hard time holding my attention? The strategies they used were not right for me.

I realized that I was not necessarily the problem when, one day, I found myself in a classroom with a teacher who held everyone's attention captive, mine included. To this day, I can still recall information I learned in her class. Why was her teaching method so effective? She used many different strategies, including ones that worked for me.

This particular teacher told stories and used props. She varied her tone of voice, and she exuded a passion for teaching. In short, she was able to engage the visual learners, the auditory learners, and the kinesthetic learners. Most of my teachers, it seemed, used only the auditory approach. This new teacher went beyond that; she used all three modalities to draw in the entire class. Her classes were fun and interactive. As a result, I never received less than 85% in her class – something I had previously been unable to achieve.

I share this story with you to demonstrate that one size does not fit all. If you have tried other programs in the past that did not produce the results you wanted, then you have not yet found the strategy that works for you. There is no failure, only positive feedback. That's why I have designed this book to include many different strategies for you to implement in order to achieve optimal, long-term results. If you have without-a-doubt belief in yourself, a "have to have it" attitude, and the right strategy, you will succeed.

Develop clarity and focus

The primary main reason most people don't get what they want in life is that they don't know exactly what they want! You may be thinking, "Of course I know what I want. I'm overweight and out of shape. Isn't it obvious? I want to lose weight and get fit." But losing weight or getting fit are neither clear nor specific enough goals to get you where you want to go.

Most people do have a clear idea of what they don't want. "I don't want to be fat." "I don't want to be broke." "I'm tired of sitting at home alone watching TV every Saturday night." But if you are constantly focusing on what you don't want, that is exactly what you are going to get. If I say to you, "don't think of the color red," what happens? You automatically think of the color red. And if you associate particular emotions with the color red, you may start to feel those emotions. What if I say, "don't think about ice cream"? You're probably on your way out the door right now to go get ice cream. Stop, right now!

What you focus on, think about, and talk about is what you are going to move toward. So focus on what you want, and be as specific as you can. For example, if you want to lose weight, what is your target weight? By what date do you want to reach your goal? What exactly are you going to do to get there? Clearly defined, compelling goals will drive your success.

The other day, I was riding in my friend's new car when we got lost. Fortunately, his car has a GPS navigational system. He gave it our exact destination, and the navigational system directed us to precisely where we wanted to go. When we arrived, I turned to him and said, "Isn't the navigational system a great metaphor for life?" "How is that?" he asked. "Your mind is like the GPS device," I explained, "Give it a clear destination, and it will go to work for you, guiding you to the very thing you want to achieve."

If you don't give the navigational system in your car a precise destination, it will not be able to direct you to where you want to go. Your mind works the same way. You must give the mind a clearly defined outcome in order to achieve your goal. Be specific about where you want to go in life, and your mind will help get you there.

Visualize success

Now that you have described in detail what you want to achieve, you must be able to visualize it. Imagine you have achieved your ideal, healthy weight. How does your body look? What is your new life like? How do you feel? Make the image in your mind as real as possible. You must have a vivid and detailed picture in your mind of what success looks like for you.

Now hold this picture of the new you in your mind as often and for as long as possible. The brain cannot distinguish the difference between something you see with your eyes and an image you create in your brain. So as you visualize your goal, your mind will begin to accept this as real, and it will strive to make your physical reality match what it "sees".

Next, find and cut out a picture of a body that looks exactly the way you would like yours to look. Choose a picture of a body that has a similar structure to yours. If you are tall with broad shoulders, for example, don't choose a picture of a short, fine-boned body. Better still, find two pictures. Place one in a prominent spot where you will see it every day, and carry the other one with you wherever you go. When you find yourself heading for a fast food drive-thru, stop and pull out the picture. Using this technique will help your goal become even more firmly embedded in your mind.

It does not matter at this point how you are going to achieve your end result. The important thing is that you be able to see in clear detail exactly what your desired outcome looks like. As you will soon discover, the how will start to take care of itself.

Don't get derailed

When you were a baby, you knew exactly what you wanted, and you were very insistent about it. When you were hungry, for example, you would cry until you were fed. In a sense, you were pursuing a specific goal, loudly and without inhibition, until you got exactly what you wanted.

Then you learned to crawl, and fueled by curiosity, you would crawl around a room towards all the things that intrigued you the most. Never did you hear a little voice in your head that said, "You can't have that!" You were still clear on exactly what you wanted, and went after it.

As we get older, we begin to hear negative messages that inhibit us in the pursuit of our goals. "Don't touch that!" "Eat everything on your plate, whether you like it or not." "Life isn't easy." "You can't have everything you want just because you want it." "Money is the root of all evil." "Can't you think of anybody but yourself?" This conditioned thinking becomes embedded in the subconscious mind and impacts our ability to set and achieve goals without us even being aware of it.

Realize that these thoughts are nothing but other people's beliefs. Be careful not to take them on and automatically accept them as true. We will work more in-depth with questioning your beliefs later. For now, just remember that you have the power to choose what you believe.

We may also unwittingly take on other people's goals as our own. People often pursue things that they don't truly want for themselves, just to please someone else. Did you earn a business degree because that's what your parents wanted you to study? Did you get a "real" job instead of pursuing your dream to be an actor? Sometimes the influence is more subtle. We fall into a "pack mentality". Maybe you don't start your own business because everyone else in your circle of friends has a "traditional" job. Or maybe everyone in your family is overweight and inactive, so it's easier for you to stay that way too.

Do not allow yourself to get derailed on the way to your dreams. You must take control over yourself, and decide exactly what you want, and who you want to become. It's time to stop making other people's needs and desires more important than yours, and make your life your own.

Stick with it!

I often see people adopt a new strategy and come close to achieving results, but they lose patience and quit. They may start a new diet or try out a new fitness program for only a week, then decide, "This doesn't work!" Remember, the excess weight did not come on overnight; it's not going to come off overnight either. To achieve results takes repetition over time. Commit to using your new strategies long enough for them to begin to work. Once you see even a tiny bit of success, you will be excited and motivated to stick with it.

How many things have you enthusiastically started, but then let slide over time? Anyone can start something, but the real winners are the ones who stick with it. The people who get the rewards in life are the ones with the staying power to achieve their goals. Think about people who are in great shape. They keep on following through, day in and day out, and they get results.

How often do you hear about someone's great new business idea that has the potential to make them rich? The average person actually has three great ideas a day. That's like holding three winning lottery tickets in your hand every day! But the ones who actually follow through on their ideas are few and far between. Follow-through is critical to your success.

I can give you every strategy I know in this book, but you must put those strategies into play, and follow through. If you don't follow through with your new personal program for weight loss success, you will get exactly the same results you always have in the past. You will have the roadmap you need, but you will be no closer to your destination. One year from today, you will think the same, look the same, and be in exactly the same place you are now. It's all up to you. You have the power to transform your life. So take action right now!

Action steps

Decide what you want

Write out your health and fitness goals. Be as specific as you can.

_____

_____

_____

_____

_____

_____

Do something different

Most of us keep doing the same things we have always done, and expect different results.

What three things can you do differently today that will help you achieve your weight loss goals?

_____

_____

_____

_____

_____

_____

Reprogram your brain

Repeating positive affirmations daily will motivate you, and help reprogram neural pathways in the brain to create new ways of thinking. Psychologists say it can take up to twenty-one days to rewire a neural pathway. The more you repeat your affirmations, with vivid imagery and strong positive emotions, the sooner they will go to work for you. Here are three examples of positive affirmations:

I am developing a strong and attractive body.

I am creating a body I enjoy and love.

I am full of energy and enjoy great health.

Now write three of your own. Carry them with you, and hang them up where you can see them every day.

_____

_____

_____

Visualization

Spend five or ten minutes creating a vivid picture in your mind of the new you. Hold this picture in your mind while you feel the emotions; feel how great it feels to be you. If this doesn't come naturally to you, then "borrow" the emotion from another time in your life when you were highly successful.

NOTES:

CHAPTER TWO
The Key To Reshape Your Body With Ease

The keys to success are taking action, having a follow-through attitude, having the resolve to stick to something with total belief in yourself, and having the right strategy. To help you develop the right strategy, I am sharing with you all the knowledge on the market today about weight loss, spanning over 250 books, and countless interviews, articles, and seminars. Thousands of hours of research have been put into this book to pinpoint with exacting accuracy why some people get lasting results from their weight loss programs while others are caught up in a whirlwind cycle of gaining and losing. If you follow this book, you will get the results you are seeking. I have designed a system and a strategy that will work for anyone; you just have to make the commitment to change once and for all.

All of the people I have worked with who have successfully achieved their ideal, healthy weight and maintained it have one thing in common. As a matter of fact, all 250 autobiographies I have read about successful people confirm that they have all done this one thing to get where they are today. And that one thing is to set goals.

The late motivational speaker, Jim Rohn, once said, "I find it fascinating that most people plan their vacations with better care than they plan their lives. Perhaps it's because escape is easier than change." To be successful, you must understand the power of goal-setting, and master this skill.

Unfortunately, most of us have heard so much talk about goal-setting that we say to ourselves, "Please don't talk to me about goal-setting! I already know everything there is to know about it." Be careful not to get caught up in that trap! The most dangerous words in the English language—words that will hold you back from success in all areas of your life—are the words, "I know that."

If you're not getting the weight loss results you want right now, following a goal-setting system is crucial. You must practice the basics over and over again. Repetition is the mother of mastery. And what differentiates people who keep their weight off from those who don't is self-mastery. They have learned to become the master of themselves and the master over their weight. They do not set goals for one month, two months, or three months and then stop; it has become a part of their daily routine.

Create a new habit

When some of my clients have an urge to go out and eat crappy food, they grab their goal-setting workbook and start writing in it. By grabbing their workbook instead of food, they break the old pattern and create a new habit. Every time I teach goal-setting, I set some new goals for myself. So don't take it for granted and say, "I already know this stuff on goal-setting." If you're not living it, you don't know it. Let me say it one more time: If you're not living it, you don't know it!

So let's break through those habits from the past and start to look at the world in a whole new way, a way that helps you understand that the basics have to be practiced every day. You have committed to do whatever it takes to succeed. Just because you have not succeeded in the past does not mean you cannot succeed this time. This is a whole new fresh start. Get excited about doing the basics daily, taking those small steps toward achieving your weight goal, because in the end, your reward will be massive. You will become a healthy, in shape, happy, excited, vibrant person who loves life.

You're probably wondering why goals are so important. Why do we need them to be a part of our lives? Why must they become a daily habit? Napoleon Hill once said, "A goal is just a dream with a deadline." Goals give us meaning and direction. Goals shape us as individuals, and they shape our lives.

We all have goals; the problem is, most people have very poorly-formed goals. A goal should engage your emotions and incite you to take action. Goals that are compelling give you the motivation to take off the weight, and keep it off once and for all. Goals can help you to become the person you have always wanted to be, and have the body you have always wanted. If your goals are set properly and are crystal clear, you will have the power to change your weight, your body, your emotions, and your life.

How to be smarter than Harvard graduates

Mark McCormack, in his book, What They Don't Teach You at Harvard Business School, tells of a Harvard study conducted between 1979 and 1989. The graduates of the MBA program were asked, "Have you set clear, written goals for your future and made plans to accomplish them?" It turned out that only three percent of the graduates had written goals and plans. Thirteen percent had goals that were not in writing. A full 84 percent had no specific goals at all, aside from getting out of school and enjoying the summer. Ten years later, in 1989, the researchers interviewed the members of that class again. They found that the 13 percent who had goals that were not in writ- ing were earning, on average, twice as much as the 84 percent of students who had no goals at all. But most surprisingly, they found that the 3 percent of graduates who had clear, written goals when they left Harvard were earning, on average, 10 times as much! The only differ- ence between the groups was the clarity of the goals they had set for themselves when they graduated. If this study does not give you the motivation to get off your butt, write your goals down daily, and review them, then I don't know what will!

I hope by now you can see the importance of having goals and writing them down. Do you want to join the three percent of the most successful people in life? Or do you want to act like the average Harvard graduate? I know that, for myself, writing down my goals has transformed my life, and it can transform yours too.

I set goals on a daily basis now. It's a habit. One night, I had just finished writing my goals. I crawled into bed, turned out the light, pulled the covers over me, and then it occurred to me that I had forgotten to brush my teeth. I realized that goal-setting was now at least as important to me as brushing my teeth. I knew in my heart, that was a true sign of success.

Of all the goals I have written down that have since become my reality, three experiences stand out the most to me. When I decided to stop using drugs, I took two full days to write out my goals and design plans for how I was going to achieve them. Second, I set an objective to find millionaires to mentor me to become a motivational speaker known around the world for helping thousands of people change their lives. Third, I set the goal to lose the extra 65 pounds I had gained, and keep it off.

When I set these goals, I had no idea how I was going to get there. At the time, some of these goals were well above my level of ability or talent. But there is a principle known to every religious man and woman, no matter what religion or god one worships, and that is the power of having absolute faith. I knew that if I could frame my goals in a way that got me excited, no matter how impossible it seemed that I could reach them, I would figure out a way to make them happen. Even if right then it seemed impossible, I would pull it off. I asked myself, "What do I want right now? What do I have to do to make it happen?"

When it came to my weight, I described the person I wanted to be in very specific detail. I wrote 10 pages about the body I wanted, how I felt inside, my level of confidence, my emotions, my energy level. I wrote about how my spouse would look at me and say, "You have a great body," how I felt in those smaller jeans, and my overall health. Eighty percent of those goals that I wrote down have become reality.

I credit a lot of my success strictly to writing down my goals daily. No doubt, there were days when I would find myself off track, but by reviewing my goals, I would get right back on. I might miss the gym or my exercise routine, or go out and cheat a little on a chocolate bar, but thanks to my goal-setting, I never strayed so far away from my goal of losing 65 pounds that I did not achieve it and keep the weight off.

Define and write your future

You have to make your goals compelling enough so they are exciting. You don't need to know how you are going to get there at this point; just get them down on paper. I am going to show you how to get there with the strategy I have for you to follow. The truth is, I don't think anyone really knows how this thing called "goal-setting" actually works, but things just start to happen. They magically appear, or in your case, the fat will magically disappear. When you write things down, something happens; you become the author of your own story.

Anybody can set goals, but you must define why you want that goal. Knowing exactly why you want it is critical to the outcome. Think about this: whatever goal you set is going to define the kind of person you become. That's why it's really important to know why you are doing it when you set a goal.

The biggest problem with goal-setting

The biggest problem with goal-setting is that people take it for granted. They think, "I know that stuff." But are you getting the results in your life that you want? Most people are not. People get the New Year's bug: "It's a new year and I am going to set a goal." But then they don't even look at it until the following New Year's. Is this you? The problem is, people do not set goals on a constant basis. Take exercise. New Year's comes around, everyone joins a gym, and three months later the only people who are still at the gym are the ones who had memberships before New Year's. Don't let this be you.

Experts say you need willpower. Wrong, you need staying power. Many people set a goal and when they don't achieve it right away, they set a new one. They have no staying power, or they take their goals way too lightly. You need commitment and persistence to create something new in your life.

Poof! It's magic after all

Realize that anything you can think of, you can achieve. I am asking you to come from a place of belief, and watch what you can make your reality. Have you ever heard the saying, "Thoughts become things."? What we consistently focus on becomes our reality. What we think, we manifest. That's why goal-setting is so important. It keeps your thoughts consistently focused on what you want.

Remember how I get off track and then I get back on again? The ability to get back with the program is all about goal-setting. You can't just set one goal, then never look at it again, and expect to get results. You need to look at your most important goals daily, weekly, and monthly to make them your reality. The power comes from consistently reviewing them on a daily basis. I truly believe the more you focus on something, the quicker you will start to experience it. Focus on enjoying exercise, and you will start to experience good health.

Think about this: when you set a goal, you're really saying to your mind, at both the conscious and unconscious levels, "I am not happy where I am right now." You start to notice the difference between where you are right now and where you want to be. Your brain says, "I am just not satisfied. There has to be more out there. I am not satisfied with my weight. I am not satisfied with losing weight, and then a year later gaining it back and then some. I am not satisfied with leaving my health to chance anymore."

It is sometimes said that success actually holds us back. Have you ever lost weight, reached your goal, and then gained all the weight back? What happened? You became too comfortable. You stopped doing all the things that got you there in the first place, so your success actually put you right back to where you were in the past. For a lot of people, success is a trap. They become successful, and start to party and eat the nights away.

Failing is not necessarily a bad thing. See it as an opportunity to change your beliefs and behaviors. When you're failing, that's when it is time to set some goals and achieve them. There is real power in using the things that you don't want in your life to push you toward the things you do want. In goal-setting, we must demand more from ourselves. When we clearly define what we want and start to demand more from ourselves, it starts to give us the motivation we need to follow through. Your brain says, "Okay, I realize that I am not already there, so I better find the drive and the means to get there."

Look at demanding more from yourself as a tool to take you to the next level. When I decided I was going to lose 65 pounds, I did not just say, "Okay, I am going to lose this weight." I sat down and figured out why I was doing it. I came up with reasons, like needing an abundance of energy so I could achieve some massive goals I had set for myself. If I did not have enough fuel, then eventually, I would sputter to a halt. To have an abundance of energy, I had to exercise at least six days per week for the next year, and never miss a day. After a year, I might go back and re-evaluate my goals. But I linked having more energy to being able to achieve my financial goals, change other people's lives, and be more effective when speaking on stage. I linked it to being there for my friends, and contributing to the world. As you can see, I had a lot of motivation.

Accountability

One of the techniques I teach is accountability. When I told people what I was going to do, I asked them to hold me accountable to my weight loss and fitness goals. I demanded more of myself. Once I told everyone, I had no way of turning back. So use the act of sharing your commitments with certain people as part of your strategy. Whatever it takes to achieve your goals, whatever it takes to get you to follow through and create results, do it.

I hope I have made it clear to you that you need a strong enough why to get yourself to take action and follow through. When I am using the why technique to help me achieve my goals, I make a list of positive reasons and a list of negative reasons. Let me give you an example of a positive reason: I am going to exercise every day because I know I will have more energy, and if I have more energy, that will help me grow my business. Now here is an example of a negative reason I use to push me forward: I ask myself, "Why would my life be worse if I did not exercise?" My answers? I would not have the energy to do business an extra two hours a day. I could end up having a heart attack or getting diabetes. And my emotions will not stay as positive throughout the day. The human brain works in mysterious ways. Sometimes we get more motivated by using the negative to push us forward rather than always using the positive.

Remember that you can change your goals at any time. The fact is, things change in our lives. Just because you picked a goal at one time does not mean you can't go back and re-evaluate that goal. I have people set goals every four months, and review them twice per month. I have them review their top goals daily. It's that kind of repetition that will keep you on track so you can achieve the outcomes you desire.

Why some people set goals and others don't

For a long time, I was interested in finding out why some people set goals and others have no goals at all. Why is it that most people have heard of the importance of goal-setting, but very few take advantage of these simple, proven techniques to achieve dreams? Why are more people not setting goals? These questions led me on a passionate journey to uncover the answers. The first clue I uncovered confirmed my prediction that people do not think goal-setting is that important. Of all the hundreds of people I talked with, the most successful ones were the people who said, "I set goals every day." The unsuccessful people would say things like, "I don't believe in setting goals," "I don't have the time," "It doesn't work," and so on.

The people who were eating healthy, exercising, and following their plan all had clearly written goals. The majority of people who were overweight had no clear goals at all. Some could tell me their goals, but they had never written them down. The wealthiest people also had clearly written goals, and reviewed them daily. Those who were broke had no written goals at all. I could clearly see a pattern. The successful ones took goal-setting very seriously. It was a daily routine, just like eating and brushing their teeth.

I came to the conclusion that if you don't write your goals down daily, you're not going to live as long, you're not going to be as successful, and you're not going to be as happy. How can you be when you have poor health? Setting goals will have more of an effect on your life than any other skill. Look around you. How many of your friends or family members have clarity and commitment to their goals? Don't follow the crowd. Step up and become a leader of yourself, others, and the world.

Lack of knowledge

Another reason I discovered that people don't set goals is they simply do not know how. You can earn a degree from a leading university without ever receiving one hour of instruction in how to set goals. Even worse, some people think they have goals, when in reality what they have is a series of wishes or dreams, like "be healthy", "make a lot of money", and "have a great family". But these are not goals at all. They are merely outcomes that everybody in society wishes for. We can all sit and daydream, but a goal, and a wish or dream are not one and the same. A goal is clear, specific, and written. It can quickly and easily be described to another person, and you can measure your progress.

Fear of failure

The third reason people don't set goals is fear of failure. Many people sabotage themselves by not setting goals at which they might fail. Every time you go on a new weight loss program and fail, it chips away at your faith in yourself. You start thinking to yourself, "Why even try again? I fail at this every time. There's just no point." But remember what I talked about in the first chapter. You did not fail; you just did not have the right strategy. With the right strategy, anybody can succeed at anything.

Throughout your journey in life you're going to have to confront many fears. Fear is a natural thing. Whenever you start a new program, a new career, or a new relationship there is usually fear. The sad thing is that most people let fear stop them from taking action and achieving their dreams. Do not let fear stop you from having the body you deserve, and the long, healthy life you deserve. In fact, don't let fear stop you from having anything that you desire in life.

Some people will do anything to avoid the uncomfortable feeling of fear. Take a look at yourself and be totally honest. Is this you? If you are one of those people who lets fear run your life, you run the biggest risk of not achieving what you want in life. Successful people experience fear too, but keep taking action until they get what they want. They understand what Susan Jeffers suggests in her book when she says, "Feel the fear and do it anyway."

Dispel your fears

I like how some psychologists refer to the word fear: Fantasized Experiences Appearing Real. We create fear in our minds before a negative outcome even exists. Our own insecurities can turn our drive to be slim and svelte into complacency. Of course we don't want to pursue our goals after we have created scary stories in our heads where our worst fears come to life. If I followed these thought processes, I would probably not come out of my room all day long. Rather than pursue a healthier life, I would watch my bulges grow.

I know some of you are saying, "What if I am too fearful to start an exercise program because I may fail? How do I get rid of fear?" One of the quickest and most powerful ways that I know of to eliminate fear from your life is to first ask yourself what you're fearful of, and notice the picture that appears in your mind. Let me give you an example: If you think of yourself exercising, you may see yourself huffing and puffing, and hating the exercise. For some of us, it may get even more intense, as we hear certain messages that spark our insecurities. Maybe it is a spouse that used to say, "I told you there is no way you are going to stick to your exercise program."So as you create an image in your mind of yourself exercising, you suddenly hear your spouse's negative words. Now you're even more fearful of joining another fitness program.

To destroy the fear of anything in life, all you have to do is manipulate the picture. Because the brain can't tell the difference between what's real and what's vividly imagined, you can actually trick it. Picture yourself full of energy and vitality, and loving exercise. See yourself in the best shape of your life. Hear your spouse saying, "Great job! I knew you could do it." Stop right now and imagine your body changing as you begin to think more positively. It is impossible to be fearful if your brain cannot imagine you being fearful. You can now follow through with anything you set your mind to.

All successful people know what they want, and they are single-mindedly focused on achieving it. Every single day, you have the ability to draw from a great power by asking yourself why. Asking yourself why is critical to the outcome. For you to take action, follow through, and write down your goals every day, you must have that desire. You must develop an intense, burning desire to achieve your goals if you really want to make them happen. For me, to create the body I had always wanted, the mindset I had always wanted, and to attract the right type of friends into my life, I had to have that burning desire. I was already there in my mind before it even happened; it was that real to me. You must make it that real for yourself.

Power strategies

Let me give you some powerful strategies you can apply to skyrocket your rate of success. These strategies can transform your life if you take action and apply them day in and day out. Remember, repetition is the mother of mastery. So let me say that one more time: you must apply them day in and day out.

What sets millionaires apart is the ability to take action. Get into the habit of taking action and following through. Once you start to form that new pattern, your life will completely change; you will begin to excel in all areas of your life.

Personal mission statements

What is a mission statement? Why is it so important? And how do you write one?

A mission statement is very simple, yet it could be one of the most important things that you ever do in your life. Just like goal-setting, people tend to take the powerful simplicity of this strategy for granted. A mission statement is the bigger vision that you want to achieve. It is something that should never be put in a desk drawer to be pulled out later. For it to work, a mission statement has to be placed somewhere prominent where you can read it every day.

Why is a personal mission statement so important? First, if you have a personal mission statement, you do not need a New Year's resolution. I get a real kick out of New Year's – everyone scrambling to set new goals, and only three percent of people will ever stick to them. It is no wonder we fail over and over again. How can anyone expect to create a change when they have been doing the same thing over and over again throughout the year – the same habits, day in and day out, for years? The fact is, ninety-nine percent of human behavior is the same as our behavior the day before.

New Year's comes along, we set a new goal, and just expect that we can make it happen. But we have not set up the right strategy to change what we have always been doing, a strategy that focuses on our daily actions. Stop setting New Year's resolutions, and start setting daily resolutions. If you create a personal mission statement and hang it somewhere where you will see it often, you can review it every day, and it will become embedded into your unconscious mind. You will begin achieving all the goals you set out for yourself, and you will never ever make a New Year's resolution again.

I have a mission statement for my health, one for my business, one for my personal life, one for my spiritual life, one for my relationship, and one for my contribution to others. You may be thinking that seems like a lot of work. It will only take you about ten minutes to do one mission statement; that's less than an hour in total if you do all five areas of your life. I am sure you can commit to less than an hour to better your life. How committed are you to success?

Get a big piece of paper, write all of your mission statements on that one page, and hang it where you can read it every day. In less than three months, your unconscious mind will be repeating your mission statements without you having to do the work anymore. It's extremely important to be in touch with your unconscious mind. Your brain has six levels, five-sixths of which are run by the unconscious mind. Those who tap into this resource will produce greater results than those who don't.

I remember the day I was writing out my health and fitness mission statement. I had just ended a three-year relationship. I got up that morning, looked in the mirror, and said to myself, "Where did this extra 65 pounds of fat come from?" For the first time in my life, I had let myself go. It really seemed like it just happened overnight. I remember feeling ripped off as I thought, "But I have written a mission statement for my health goals. This stuff must not work!

Everything I have learned is useless." But then I started digging a little deeper. And as I did, my unconscious mind blurted out, "How do you expect me to help you when your mission statement has been stuck away in a drawer and not reviewed for over seven months? You're asking me to guide you but you're giving me nothing to direct you with."

Hmmmm, my unconscious mind had a point. It said to me, "Shane, repetition is the mother of mastery; out of sight, out of mind." Yes, now I remembered. When I was in great shape, I had my mission statement posted where I could see it, and I read it twice a day, when I awoke in the morning and right before bed at night. It was like the map for my unconscious mind; I gave it direction, and it took me to exactly where I wanted to go. We were a team, working together. If you want to be one hundred percent aligned within yourself, you must have the unconscious mind and conscious mind working as a whole. That day, I took my very first step toward taking off the 65 pounds of unwanted fat I had around my belly. I sat down and wrote my mission statement. I picked a place to hang it where I could see it every day, and I read it morning and night.

Once you read your mission statement so many times that it gets embedded in your unconscious mind, you can be walking down the street past an ice cream shop, and the next thing you know, your teammate, the unconscious mind, steps in to play the game. It no longer sits on the sidelines. Suddenly, you're hearing your mission statement all around you, and I guarantee it's not directing you into the ice cream shop. Your conscious mind may have been tackled by the temptation, but your unconscious mind has a different game plan, one that does not include ice cream.

Actually, it's just the feeling that ice cream gives you that you are addicted to. We get addicted to certain emotional states. So as you go to open the door to the ice cream shop, hoping to get that quick, good feeling from the ice cream, your unconscious mind brings you back to the reality of your long-term goal. It will not let you be subjected to the temptation of immediate gratification because it knows that long-term success is much more rewarding. All of a sudden, your conscious mind wakes up, and you're no longer walking around in a trance like most of society. Your conscious mind decides to work together with your unconscious mind, and you make the decision to walk right by the ice cream shop. As you get farther away, you feel a sense of control and personal power from within. If you do this enough times, you will form a completely new habit. That's the power of having a mission statement work for you. You're constantly reinforcing your mind with the positive thoughts of exactly what you want. What you think about and talk about is what you're going to get.

Henry David Thoreau once said, "If one advances confidently in the direction of his dreams...he will meet with a success unexpected in common hours." This is exactly what happens when you read your mission statement morning and night. You will start to meet with success in the most unexpected hours. That's really how powerful a mission statement can be. If you do this repetitively, things will just magically start to happen. A mission statement will keep you going in the right direction until you achieve your goal. Most of us discredit the power of goal-setting. If you want to join the high achievers of the world, then it's time to start setting goals – daily, weekly, and monthly; not just every New Year's, but throughout the year.

Be specific

Your goals must be very specific. Part of the reason we write down and examine our goals is to create a set of instructions for our unconscious mind to carry out. Your unconscious mind is a very efficient tool. It cannot determine right from wrong, and it does not judge. Make sure your goals are specific and stated in a positive manner. A representation stated in the positive motivates the mind more than one stated in the negative. The truth is, the human mind does not process a negative.

Let's take health, for example: If you say, "I am not going to gain any more weight," your brain automatically hears the word gain and will direct you to the very thing you don't want, and that is to gain weight. "I will take care of my health," would be a better way to state it. Or state your goal in the present tense – for example, "I am at my ideal, healthy weight of 150 pounds," – as though you have already achieved it. This will create an image in your mind of you already at your ideal, healthy weight, and direct you to that exact thing. Just think what kind of empowering state that will put you in. When you're in a positive state – feeling confident, happy, and grateful – it's a lot easier for you to achieve your outcomes.

Rewrite your goals daily

Every morning when you wake up, take several minutes to rewrite your goals. This step is one of the most important in setting goals that you actually achieve. If you do this every morning and every night before you go to sleep, you can trick your unconscious mind into believing that you already have the things you desire.

Here's an example of a written goal from one of my clients:

I am taking exciting steps to achieve my ideal, healthy weight of 135 pounds in a fun and motivating manner. I will do this by going to the gym five times per week. I will prepare and choose to eat only healthy foods. I love the food that makes me thin.

Her goal was very specific. At the time, she weighed 190 pounds. She is now down to her desired weight of 135 pounds. She says that there is no way she could have done this without writing down her goal every day. By writing down her goal in a positive manner, she started to feel that she was already there. Every day this statement kept her working towards her goal. She admits that at first she did not believe this could work, but she just kept with it, writing it down day after day, week after week. There were days when she felt like not exercising, but by writing down her goal, something inside her would say, "You have to go." That's the power of the unconscious mind. She now enjoys a very rewarding, healthy life.

I personally use this strategy every night before I go to bed and every morning when I awaken. It only takes about two or three minutes. How about setting your alarm five minutes earlier so you can set yourself up for success for the rest of your life? One of the major reasons people are not getting the results they want is because they're not following through. It is so important that you make a decision to do this today. Turn off your phone, turn off the TV, and go to a place where the kids can't interrupt you. Let people know that you can't be disturbed; that you're ready to create a new and rewarding future; that you're going to use all your drive, motivation, and skill to make your life the way you truly want it to be.

People often say to me, "Shane, I'm just lazy." It's not that you're lazy; you just don't have goals that get you really excited. To live a long, healthy life and really, I mean, really, enjoy life should get you excited. Realize that right now you're about to create a new future, with a new body and more energy, a future that can make a major difference in the quality of your life.

You're not just writing words down on a piece of paper for the fun of it. You may not know exactly when and how this is all going to happen, but if you have strong enough reasons, you will find or create a way. You will acquire that unstoppable motivation. People routinely exclaim, "Shane, you're always so motivated, you're bouncing off the walls most of the time." I have created enough compelling reasons why I want change in my life. My reasons for changing my life are so strong, and get me so excited, that I will do anything to achieve my goals.

Don't be afraid to set big goals

The kinds of results you will generate are going to be amazing. We have so many more capabilities within us than we know. When you get to that level where your brain actually believes that your goal is already real, things just start to happen. You very often get to that goal in a very short period of time. I know this may sound metaphysical, but this principle has created positive change in thousands of people's lives, including my own.

I want you to do something for me right now; even if you don't want to, please just humor me. I want you to put yourself into a state of mind of absolute belief, of total faith that you can have the body you deserve, the life you deserve. As a matter of fact, you can have anything you truly want if you have total faith. I want you to get into that state.

Go back and remember when you were a child, and pretend it's Christmas Eve. A child has no problem creating a list of exactly what they want. They will tell Santa precisely what they want — and the exact day they expect to get! If you ask them, "What do you want for Christmas?" they'll respond, "I want a bike; not just any bike, a blue bike with bells on it. And a helmet to go with it; not just any helmet, this specific one with this exact design on it. And then how about we throw in a bike for you, too, and for all the other kids?" As an adult, you think this is a fantasy world. But with that kind of thinking, you will be lucky to get any kind of bike at all! You must come from a mindset of absolute belief, placing no limitations on yourself.

Track your progress

Set small goals that will lead into big goals, and write dates for your monthly goals. This will keep you focused and on track. If your goal is to lose 48 pounds in six months, write down how much you want to lose monthly – it may be eight pounds per month – and by what date. Measure your progress daily. There is great power in tracking your success. You can clearly see if you're moving in the right direction or not.

Setting objectives that are observable is very impor-tant in the goal-setting process. When I say observable, I am talking about including a description of the behavioral change that you want to observe in your goal. By doing this, you can see when you're achieving your goal, because you will start to see a specific, observable change. If you find it hard to describe an observable change, think from another person's perspective. What would another person looking in on my life identify as a change? For example, a behavioral change might be exercising five days a week, and as a result, your energy is extremely high and you don't go in and out of depressed states. Becoming observant of the changes you're making or not making is going to be a critical determining factor in your success.

We have covered a lot of strategies for creating the power to achieve goals. I hope you realize just how impor-tant it is to set and keep goals. Remember that only three percent of people who achieve their goals write them down and review them.

If you invest $200,000 in a business, and a wise mentor tells you that you need a business plan to decrease your chances of losing your money, will you go create a business plan? Will you write a mission statement for your new business? Of course you will. There is no way that you would even consider not doing it. You would say, "There is no way I am losing my $200,000!"

Why not do the same with your body and your health? It's much more important than the $200,000. This will determine how many good, healthy years you add to your lifespan. You see, the $200,000 does not matter. It's just money; big deal! You can lose all of your money, and then work to make it all back again. If you lose your life to poor health, you don't get another shot. So my advice to you is work as hard for great health as you do to support yourself and your family.

One final note: remember to enjoy the present as you work your way toward your future goals. One mistake I find many people make is that they are so busy striving for their goals (or they don't have any goals) that they're consistently getting stressed out and frustrated, and feeling that their life is going nowhere. Just be happy with the person you are right now and enjoy every moment. Success comes from taking those starting steps, just like a child learning to walk, and never giving up until you reach your goals. If you put this plan into place, you will reap the rewards. Remember, you're conditioning yourself for a new and better way to live, a way that's creating unstoppable power within.

Action Steps

Have someone hold you accountable.

Pick one person and tell them your goals. Check in with them twice per week.

Who is that person? (Call them now!)

Create a personal mission statement.

Use a big piece of paper to write all of your mission statements on. Start with your weight loss mission statement. Write down your weight loss goal, and make sure it is specific and measurable. Hang it where you can read it every day.

Example:

> *I am taking exciting steps to achieve my ideal, healthy weight of 135 pounds in a fun and motivating manner. I will do this by going to the gym five times per week. I will prepare and choose to eat only healthy foods. I love the food that makes me thin.*

Your weight loss goal:

_____

_____

_____

_____

Rewrite your goals daily

Every morning when you wake up, and again before you go to bed, take several minutes to rewrite your goals. Put a notebook beside your bed and get into the habit of doing this daily. Do not put any limitations on yourself; if you can think it, you can create it!

CHAPTER THREE
Behavioural Changes To Forever Weight Loss

We all seek the motivation, insight and wisdom to turn our goals into reality. Without the right motivation, as we get closer and closer to our long-sought goals, they may turn into a mirage. The wrong motivation is why many weight loss plans spiral into a cycle of yo-yo dieting.

The key to a lifetime of better health lies in understanding Kirstie Alley's fat-to-riches story. The more weight she gains, the more money she makes for losing it. Here she is again on a reality TV show; another weight loss gig, another cool $10 million. Are the negative health effects of yo-yo dieting – nutritional deficiencies, emotional and mental stress, and potential organ damage – worth all the money in the world? Kirstie is Big Life proof that we need the right motivation to change our lives. As I watch Kirstie spend her money on her reality TV show, I want to give her a big, comforting hug, and help her explore her real problems.

The promise I make to you in this chapter is to show you how to face the real challenges affecting your health, weight and quality of life by helping you find that true motivation. The challenges we face require only one thing, and that is that we learn to act differently. Every motivational speaker, weight loss guru, or expert can offer solutions, but the real change comes when people act differently and change their behavior. Whether you want to lose five pounds or 150 pounds, if you follow the steps in this chapter, you will start to act differently and your weight will change. You will no longer think and act like an overweight person, and you will achieve your desired weight.

By the end of this chapter you will:

- Discover behaviors that have been holding you back from years of success

- Develop completely new behaviors and a new way of doing things

- Start to look at yourself and the world in a whole new light

How do we change behaviors? According to the man who inspired the world to make better products, you need to be a master of improving the quality of your life. In the 1950s, American management consultant W. Edwards Deming went to Japan to find out why the Japanese built better cars. Deming learned that by empowering the worker on the factory floor, everything from cars to TVs could be made better, cheaper and faster. The same principle holds true for building better health. Deming put it best: "It's not enough to do your best; you must know what to do, and then do your best."

It's not enough to want to lose weight. Before you can lose weight, you first must decide why you are doing it. Most people have no clue why they want something. They may think they do, but they really don't.

What would be a strong enough why to motivate you to achieve your ideal healthy weight for the rest of your life? To be full of energy and vitality? To produce strong, healthy cells? Think about it. The only reason that you follow through with anything in your life is because you have found a compelling enough why.

Once you have found this motivation, nobody will have to tell you to get up early in the morning or stay up late at night to fit in a workout. Nobody will have to tell you to go that extra step to achieve all the success you have been aching for in your life. Nobody will have to tell you because you will have a strong enough why. Even if what you're doing is outside your comfort zone, you will not hesitate to break right through your fear and come out the other side in the winner's circle.

I ask my clients, "Do you want to be in great shape?" "Of course," they typically say, "That's a dumb question, Shane." But what is really behind that desire? You don't just want to be in great shape. Maybe you want to have more energy, to feel great, to look hot, to live longer, to be able to play with your children or grandchildren without getting tired, or to have a fantastic attitude.

This is the why that really drives you, that gets you so excited and emotionally charged that you will do anything to achieve your goal. When you know exactly what you want and you have a strong enough why, your newfound motivation will literally light a fire inside of you.

In search of your why

When I acquired my first and closest mentor six years ago, he sat me down in his office and asked me some important, life-changing questions. I was young, and so excited, and telling him all my dreams and goals with so much enthusiasm. On and on I gushed until he cut me off mid-sentence. "Shane, stop." "What do you mean, stop?" I implored, "I have so much more to tell you."

"Shane, listen closely," he said, "You understand business, and you're one of the most motivated people I have ever met in my life. It's just a matter of time before you're at the top." His comments got me even more excited. Here was a man who makes over one hundred million dollars a year telling me that I was going to make it big.

In those days, I had trouble controlling my excitement and keeping my mouth shut. "Come on, I have this great idea. Just let me tell you," I said.

I am glad he had so much patience with me. "Shane, listen closely," he repeated. "Why do you want success?"

I thought, "What a dumb question. I'm wasting my time here." How could this guy have made one hundred million dollars and ask why I want to be successful? I had the cockiest attitude back then. I stood up and said, "To make one hundred million dollars, just like you." And he said, in a calm voice, "Shane, go home and think about this question for the next two weeks and then come back and see me."

"What, so I can come back and say the same thing?" I thought, "What kind of mentorship is this? I thought he was going to teach me how to make lots of money!"

"I'll see you in two weeks," he said. I stormed out of his office, fire coming out of my ears.

I went home and pondered the question for a week, still not coming up with anything other than my strong desire to make one hundred million dollars. The following week, the answers finally started to come. I had many reasons to make one hundred million dollars. I could help hundreds of thousands of people live better lives. I could help them change their weight forever. I could help humanity by making the world a better place to live. I realized I wanted to become better at everything I do, and help as many people as I could overcome their challenges along the way.

"Yes," I said to myself, "It's about making the world a better place. If I could make a difference in the world and help people, how awesome would that be? It's not about me, but about helping as many people as I can. If I'm not giving, I'm not living." It was like a light bulb went on in my head, or maybe a higher power showing me why I was really here on earth.

Now I understood what my true purpose was. The commitment to helping others was now propelling me forward. I was so excited about going back to see my mentor that the night before our meeting I was like a kid on Christmas Eve. I kept looking at the clock. Is it time to get up yet? Finally, my alarm went off that morning. I jumped out of bed yelling, "Let's go help people, and make the world a better place!"

On my way to the meeting that day I was so excited, I was driving a little too fast. The next thing I know, I was pulled over by a police officer. He walked up to my window and asked, "Young man, how come you're driving so fast?"

"I'm on my way to help people and change the world, make it a better place!" I shouted, "That's why I'm here on earth!"

He took a step back, looking at me as if I were possessed. I quickly started to explain. Then, with a smirk, he said, "You have a good meeting, and drive the speed limit on your way." I never received a ticket that day.

As I walked into my mentor's office, he was sitting in his usual place behind his desk. "I got it! I know exactly why I'm here," I yelled, "It took me about a week, but I figured it out. I'm here to make one hundred million dollars. Hallelujah! I'm going to be rich! Thanks for the advice." His look was priceless.

Then I said, "Just kidding. I'm here to help people, to change the world, to make the world a better place, and to put other people before myself. I realized I can only be happy if I am helping humanity."

He stood up and looked over at me with the most disappointed look on his face. Then he slowly sat back down in his chair and shook his head with a slight air of disgust. I thought to myself, "What more can he want? What could be a better answer than that?"

"Just kidding," he said, a big grin spreading across his face. "Don't ever try to trick one of your mentors. Believe me, you won't win. They'll always get the last laugh."

"Shane," he continued, "you just found a compelling enough reason to keep you going until you reach your goal. You have a strong enough why that will keep you motivated but, more importantly, when you get there you're going to feel like you have accomplished something other than just having a large bank account balance."

With these wise words, my mentor set me off on the journey I am on today. And it is this same message that I would like to share with you. You have to have a strong enough why or you're not going to follow through on your weight loss goal. The more powerful your why, the more compelling your journey will be, and the more emotional commitment you will have attached to your goal. A strong enough why can change your weight and your life. Once you have a convincing why, you will do whatever it takes to achieve your goal. No matter what challenges, obstacles, or setbacks you face; no matter what food is put in front of you; no matter what injury or medical condition you have; no matter what, you will always find or create a way because you have a powerful enough why.

Developing behavioral flexibility

Once you have a motivating why, you then need to have the behavioral flexibility to achieve your goal. If you keep doing the same thing, you're going to keep getting the same result. If what you're doing gets you closer to your goal, then keep doing it. But if you are not getting closer to your goal, you have to be able to recognize what's working and what's not, and start doing things differently.

The problem is most people are stuck in behavioral patterns that are not taking them closer to their goals. They get set in their ways. Political leaders, for example, would make terrible weight loss consultants. So often countries remain in the same political quagmire for decades – North and South Korea, or Israel and Palestine, for example – because neither side will change their behavior.

If you have behavioral flexibility, you can keep changing and adapting to situations until you get exactly what you want. If you're in an argument with someone and you want the communication to work out for both of you, develop flexibility in your own communication and keep adapting to the other person. Eventually, you will both end up happy.

It's tough at times to change our approach because most of the time we're so used to doing things a certain way. But if you adopt an attitude of behavioral flexibility, you can change your outcomes. I can't count how many times I have had to change my course of action to get to where I am today. When I started to use this approach, my life changed dramatically. I started to become consciously aware of what was working and what was not.

Take relationships. How many people keep choosing the exact same behavior and just hoping the relationship is going to get better?

Where else in your life do you feel that you need some behavioral flexibility? Where do you feel you have been stuck in the same behavior, and if you were to change that behavior your life would completely change?

Everyone reading this book wants to lose some weight. When we're exercising and eating healthy we can literally start to see the change in our energy in weeks, days, or sometimes even hours or minutes. So as you're going along on your journey, it's really important to stop and look at what you're doing. Is what you're doing taking you closer to your weight loss goal? Or is it taking you farther away from your goal? All you have to do to have massive success with weight loss and in life is to have behavioral flexibility – notice what's working and what's not, and change your direction.

Why don't most of us have behavioral flexibility? We become too stubborn, caught up in patterns of doing things the same way. In turn, the pain of not adapting to new situations gets into our nervous system, and becomes deeply embedded into our thought patterns. We become even more stuck, choosing the same behaviors over and over, and the cycle continues. We become unconscious, not even aware of what's going on around us. If you're like most people, you face several challenges that cause you to freeze rather than fluidly adapt.

Underlying behavioral issues

Every weight loss guru is wrong. For years, they have been telling you over and over that you have a weight problem, but you don't. You have a behavioral problem. Most likely, you have not been provided with the right behavioral strategy – one that works for you – to produce lasting results. You may try one or two different behaviors and when those don't work, you label yourself a failure. You say things like, "I just can't succeed at weight loss." You surrender and move on.

Now if you were able to identify the two most vital behaviors behind your inertia, you could create everlasting change. Identifying those can create a massive amount of change for anyone. Even the most deeply ingrained problems can be solved through finding and adjusting a few high-leverage behaviors. Find these trigger points and you will start to write your own ticket for success in all areas of your life.

One must be very careful not to confuse outcome with behaviors. Experts are often focused on the outcome, not on changing the underlying behavior. Although their advice may sound good, it gives you no clear direction as to what to do. They're really saying, "You need to do something, but I'm not quite sure what you should do." Be very careful with advice from experts. If they're focusing only on the outcome, speak up and ask them to be more specific about the details on what you should do to get the results you want.

Confusing outcomes with behavior is no small issue. It can have a significant impact on your ability to create future success. Let's take a closer look at the difference.

Reprogramming behavioral patterns

You first must change your behavioral patterns. And in order to do that, you must engage in deep self-analysis to identify all the triggers that encourage you to overeat, and then change them.

Many weight loss programs only skim the surface of behavioral change. My neighbor, Molly, for example, recently dropped by for tea and relationship advice – advice on her relationship with food, that is. She had just attended a seminar on weight loss, and had been told that in order to reach her ideal healthy weight she had to establish a good relationship with healthy foods. That's it. That's what she was directed to do. She was given advice from a weight loss expert who felt he was giving clear direction on how to change behavior. In truth, she was being told to do something to develop a healthy relationship with food, but not precisely what to do. She left the seminar more confused than when she arrived.

I see many programs designed around the outcome, or that only give half the information on how to change your behavior and leave out the other half: how to create lasting change.

When we decide to start changing our behavior, the first step is to become aware of our established behavior. We want to focus on those patterns we do over and over again.

Have you ever been in the middle of looking for something and then all of a sudden you notice your brain has gone off in some other direction? Let's say you are looking for weight loss information on the Internet. You're fully focused on finding it but then you click on your favorite news site, something you do at least three times a day. This thinking starts to become established behavior, and these patterns in your brain often keep you from succeeding at the things you want to achieve. You're trying to achieve what you want – in this case, finding that new weight loss information – but you keep doing the same things over and over, and expecting different results. That's why I call it established behavior.

The key to developing positive life change is to break these habits that keep us from achieving the things we want so badly, and reprogram our patterns of behavior. We're not just going to change the old habits; we're going to replace them with something new.

How to do pattern interrupts

Think about overeating. This has become such an established behavior that the habit is ingrained in you. I know for myself, at one time I would run this pattern over and over. I had no idea that there were so many triggers inside me.

To create a new pattern, like living a healthy, vibrant life, you must first interrupt the old pattern. Let me give you a quick analogy. Every day you turn on the radio, and for years you have listened to the same host at the same time. It's almost as if he is a part of your family. Then one day you turn on the radio at the usual time and you hear a different voice, and the dreaded news that your favorite host has been replaced. Your brain thinks, "Oh, my goodness, this can't be happening. My days are never going to be the same." This experience has interrupted your pattern.

So what we want to do is interrupt all the negative mental patterns that are holding you back from living a healthy life, the ones that say, "Exercise is hard. I can't do it. I can't stick with a program."

Remember, if you failed in the past it was not you; you just did not have the right strategy. Let me stress one more time the importance of interrupting those patterns. If you interrupt any pattern enough times, you will never go back to it. This process literally takes the brain and neurologically scrambles the way it thinks. What happens when you change the code for your alarm on your house? You scramble the sequence; it can't go back to the old code. Your brain works the same way. Once you scramble the sequence in your brain, you won't go back to the old pattern. You will change the habits you have been stuck in.

To make pattern interrupts work, you must do things differently, and attach significant emotional intensity to the experience. If you follow these steps, you will never go back to that mindset again. So if I ask you to do something that's completely outside the box, go for it. Believe me, this strategy will work. Our goal is to create new habits. Come up with your own ways to create fun, outside-the-box pattern interrupts that work for you.

People often say to me, "I am ready to make a change, but when I do, it only lasts one day, a week, or a month at best." You must create a follow-through attitude. You must be willing to do whatever it takes for as long as it takes.

I used to say to myself, "I'm not going to eat any desserts this week. For the next seven days, I'm going to eliminate having desserts at the end of each meal, and I'm going to start to lose weight once and for all. I'm going to take complete control of my life. This time I'm really going to do it. I have all the willpower in the world."

I was very clear on my outcome. But you know what would happen on the third day? I would start thinking, "One little bite of dessert isn't going to hurt me. It's just one bite." I would take that one little bite, and day four would come along. Well, one little bite did not hurt me the last time. I stepped on the scale and hadn't gained an ounce. I can have one more little bite tonight. But this time one bite turned into half the dessert. It just tasted so good. Half won't hurt me; it's not the full dessert. By day seven, I am eating the full dessert, plus everybody else's.

Gaining control

So what does the word control mean? It means to have power over, or to direct something. It gives us tremendous ability to achieve results, but with less effort. We have to get control over ourselves to the extent that our brain recognizes that a dip in commitment is going to take away from all the success we want to create. Once we make a commitment, we need to be able to stick to it. We don't need to choose instant gratification over long-term success. We have to make the link that making this change is going to give us great feelings.

Think about how bad it feels to be overweight, and the prospect of continuing to live with those emotions if you don't make a change. Now think about how good it feels to be thin. You must remember those good feelings in your body; how energetic, confident, vibrant, and healthy you feel. Now tell me, can any food compare to that wholesome feeling? I don't think so. Why not think of those feelings before you eat crappy food? Feel them before you raise that fork up to your mouth with all that junk on it.

We're going to start to train your body and mind to do this. How to get control, so that when you make a choice, you're not making it based on how much food you're going to eat, but on how good you will feel putting the right foods into you. You will feel full of energy and alive.

One of the biggest obstacles is that we "should" our-selves. We should lose weight, we should take action, we should exercise, we should control our emotions. We should, we should, we should. You get my drift. Quit "should-ing" yourself. Change those "shoulds" into choices. I choose to do this for my health. I choose to do this for my weight. I choose to do this for myself. Make everything a choice instead of "shoulding" yourself every day.

Remember that the goal of this book is to make losing weight simple and easy for you. Most people drop out of programs because they're too complex, they're too overwhelming. If I made this book hard, very few people would follow through. I want you to be able to stop overeating once and for all, to get out there and really enjoy your life, be healthy and in shape, and have the body and mindset you so deserve.

If you have failed in the past, it does not mean you have failed. You just did not have the right tools to succeed. Whatever has happened in your past is over and done with. This is a new day, a new book, a new way of life. Now you'll have the right tools to be effective once and for all, and to make change fun and pleasurable. I promise you success if you apply these strategies day in and day out.

It's hard to overcome addictions. Whether it's an addiction to drugs, food, alcohol, gambling, or smoking, one of the major reasons why it's hard for people to take control is they just don't want to admit that they are addicted. It does not mean you're a bad person if you're addicted to food or anything else. That's just the behavior that you're choosing at that time. That's not really you. Any learned behavior can be unlearned with the right strategy.

So the first step is to be honest about where you're having a problem. Stop rationalizing, minimizing and excusing, and admit that there is an area of your life you really need to work on. Start today, and set yourself free. Use the strategies and techniques in this book to help you take control of yourself and create the change you're looking for, but first you must take full responsibility.

Identify a few vital behaviors

Once we become aware of the few vital behaviors we're choosing that are taking us farther away from our goals, we can replace them. Many of us do not become successful or reach our health goals because we are consistently making the same choices. We might break the old habits for a while, then we go right back to the same behaviors that were holding us back. If you have been on diet after diet after diet, this is you.

There are so many ways to change your patterns – reaching for unhealthy foods, for example – but you have to have something new to replace them with. Instead you could laugh, go exercise, drink water, listen to music, sing out loud, take a shower, or start a conversation. It has to be something you love doing, something that will keep you away from the food. Eating will only shift your focus away from your problems for a short period of time, and when the problems return, they will be that much worse. You have to create a new way of refocusing. If you add emotional intensity and fun to the new behavior, it will become linked into your nervous system. And if you keep repeating the new behavior on a consistent basis, it will become a lifelong habit.

This is by far the most critical step. If you do this step correctly, it can completely change your old, limiting behaviors for the rest of your life. Wouldn't it feel good to have a totally new way of doing things, behaviors that help support you in all your goals? Then, if you were to walk by some unhealthy food, your new response would be, "No way! You're not getting me this time. I know that being thin feels much better than being fat, much better than any food I will ever put in my mouth."

Create a repetitive pattern

The next step in adopting the new behavior is repetition. You have broken the old pattern, and you now have an opportunity to train your brain with the new one. The brain doesn't yet know what to do. The new ways of thinking and acting have to become a habit. They have to be repeated until your brain becomes conditioned. Any new behavior that you fail to repeat over and over will eventually die and you will revert to the old habit. It's really that simple. The bottom line is if you don't use something, over time the brain loses neural connections and it will just disappear.

What we're going to do next is condition your mind by getting you to repeat the new pattern over and over. Each time you do it, it will be with more emotional intensity. The higher the emotional intensity, the easier it is to condition yourself so it becomes a lifelong behavior.

One of the biggest problems is people try to make too many changes all at once. This is the wrong approach. Your brain is not equipped to handle this overload. Changing just a few vital behaviors can drive big results. Soon you will have tremendous control over your life and the health you have always deserved.

People always say they want to lose weight, but it's fat you really want to lose. I could put you on a program that helps you lose weight by losing water, but if you lose too much water, you're going to die. I could put you on a program that helps you lose weight by losing muscle, but when you lose muscle your metabolism drops and you don't burn fat effectively.

We have talked a lot about patterns, instilling new habits, and creating brand new behaviors. This is one of the most important steps you're going to learn in creating a permanent change in your weight. In fact, this will be one of the most important steps you learn to change anything in your life.

Doing it

Once you have your new pattern, you have to start doing it. Not practicing it, but doing it. Don't ever say you're going to practice. The word practice tells your brain you're not good at something. It's time now to take on an "I just do" attitude. You take never-ending, consistent action until you succeed. You do and you do and you do. That's all your brain is programmed for; you don't know any differently.

Let's explore thinking that will create your ideal body versus counterproductive thoughts. What if I say to you, "If you want to be in great shape then this is what you have to do: go to the gym five days per week."? And what if instead you decide to go only three days per week? Are you going to have better results going three days or five days? Five, of course.

So stop coming up with excuses. "I don't have time to work out because I have to take the kids to hockey practice." "My job comes first." "I have to cook dinner." "My family takes priority." This kind of thinking gets in the way of saying, "I am just going to do it."

Making excuse after excuse is a common pattern that holds people back, but you may be unaware of its strong hold on your life. You must start thinking that there are no ifs, no ands, no buts, no should haves, no could haves and no would haves. Your mantra must become "I just do." It's really that simple. You don't need to give it any more thought. You put on your shoes, you go out the door, you get to the gym and you work out. And you say to yourself over and over, "I just do, I just do," until you have a completely new behavior established.

The only advantage that really successful people have over people who are not as successful is the ability to take action. If someone is in great shape, it's because they have figured out how to go out and take action. They don't just think about it or talk about it; they do it. Similarly, a person does not become a millionaire by thinking or talking about it; they just go out and do it.

Being it

The next and last step is being it. This is when you have mastered what you're doing. You don't even realize you're doing it because you know it so well. Once you go into a state of being, you're no longer thinking the same thoughts, feeling the same feelings, producing the same brain chemicals, or being the exact same person you have always been. This is where true change happens. When you're at this stage, you do not have to consciously activate your new way of being; it's automatic.

Today, you're learning new knowledge. The problem is that people learn something new, act on it for a short time, and then say, "I know this stuff,' and move on to the next book, set of CDs, or seminar. But they don't really know it. They have not yet reached the stage of mastering it.

Being it – your new way of thinking and living – is when a skill becomes so easy you can do it with your eyes closed. It's natural and effortless. Have you ever asked someone how they do something and they say, "I am not sure, I just do it."? They have reached the stage of mastery; they are no longer doing, they are simply being.

When I started speaking, I just kept doing it and doing it until I mastered it. The first time I got up on stage, it was in front of a group of kids. When I was done, they clapped and cheered, even though I really had no idea what I was doing or saying. Then I started giving talks to people like you, and I used the same accelerated learning techniques, encouraging people to participate so they could learn more. And again, everyone clapped and cheered. I still wasn't quite sure what the heck I was doing, I was just doing it. Then I did my first corporate speech and I used the same techniques. There I was in a room full of suits and ties, and I swear they had no idea what the words playful and fun even meant. I asked a room full of guys in suits to turn to the person on their left and the person on their right and give them each a hug, and promptly discovered that they didn't fully appreciate the power of the hug. But I persevered, and they too clapped and cheered. Now, speaking is not just what I do, it has become a part of who I am.

When you start really being it, you're living it. It's like being "in the zone." All your focus is on one thing and nothing else enters your mind; you're in a state of being. You often hear of sports players who get into the zone. When a sports player is in the zone, he's focused on the here and now. When a tennis player is in the zone, as they move to hit the ball, they may be out of breath, but their bodies are full of energy and free of tension. Moving gracefully, they feel as if they're floating along, barely moving. As they play each point they don't care if they're 5-1 ahead or 0-5 behind. They put 100 percent effort into each point. By using this strategy, they become very hard to beat. It's unlikely they will lose the lead and therefore the game. When you get into the zone, like a sports player, you will feel as if every movement is effortless.

Think back and remember a time when you were in the zone, when everything seemed to be going right, and you felt as if your actions were effortless. I can remember times when I was in the zone speaking on stage. As I moved gracefully around the stage, I was completely focused on that moment. I could not hear anything around me even though the room was filled with thousands of people. Every word seemed to come out at exactly the right moment, in the right tone; every story moved the crowd. And then, the next thing I knew, my talk was coming to an end. It seemed like I had only been on stage for five minutes, but it had already been two hours. How did the time go by so fast? That's the power of being in the zone.

I also experience this state when it comes to my health

and fitness. Many times I get so absorbed in my workout that with every step I take, every weight I lift , every sit-up I do, I don't even realize that I am exercising. This is because I am just being in that moment. I am so focused on having great health and a great body, and I have done it for so long now that I don't know any differently.

Changing your behavior

Now it's time for you to take action. Follow these steps to begin transforming your life by changing one self-limiting behavior at a time.

Name your feelings

1. Find an experience in the past when you weren't performing at your best. Step back into the experience just long enough to become aware of the feelings you were having. Then name your feelings: frustrated, overwhelmed, confused, fearful, panicked, nervous, angry, or whatever that emotion may have been for you.

Dissociate from the behavior

2. Now, dissociate from the event. As you float out above yourself, watch yourself behaving the way you did at the time. As you do this, you will be gathering information, both consciously and unconsciously.

Choose your emotions

3. As you watch this movie of yourself, ask yourself what emotions you would like to be experiencing during this event. Perhaps it's happy, centered, calm, excited, motivated, persistent, loving, or sensual. Choose whatever that emotion would be.

See yourself doing the new behavior

4. Keeping the positive emotion in your mind, see yourself choosing different behaviors that will give you the feelings you want. Pick three new actions that elicit positive feelings. Make one of them playful and outrageous. Run through variations and revise them. Take some time to do this properly.

Associate with the new behavior

5. Step into the first new behavior you chose. See yourself acting that way and become aware of your new feelings. Make sure you're associated with the event; that is, seeing it through your own eyes. How much emotional intensity does this new view of yourself create inside you?

   Now set this behavior aside and step into your second choice. Experience what this choice is like through your own eyes. Become aware of the feelings you're experiencing. Check the intensity of this second emotion.

Compare both new behaviors

6. Which one of these two new emotions is the most intense? Pick the strongest one and set it aside. Once you have decided which new emotion is the strongest, hear an excited voice with lots of enthusiasm saying, "This is the one I am going to do."

Program the new behavior

7. Now program this new behavior so that it's automatic. Think of an external trigger you will encounter as the situation begins. For example, for working out, the trigger could be seeing the exercise machines you're going to use. If it's talking with an angry spouse, the trigger could be hearing the an-

gry words and tone. Then, put yourself right there in the situation behaving in the positive new way you have chosen, feeling the new feelings.

Psychologists often say, "It takes months to unlearn a habit. This is false. You can replace any habit with a more desirable one quickly. If you find a better way to drive to work, how many times does it take before you stop automatically turning down the old street? Not many!

Remember, it's the behaviors that we have been engaging in for many years that are holding us back from success. Shifting them will turn your life in the direction of happiness and success.

Anchoring

So far, I have given you several techniques to change your behavior. Now I am going to teach you how to get anchored to that behavior.

What do I mean by anchoring?

Let me first define an anchor. It's any external stimulus that triggers an internal response, influencing your state of mind. The stimulus could be a word, object, person, or sensory input. The state and the stimulus become neurologically linked. Then any time the stimulus is provided, the state reoccurs.

The associations created can be either positive or negative. A positive anchor creates a positive response; a negative anchor evokes a negative response. An example of a positive anchor might be hearing your favorite song on the radio. You hear this song, and suddenly you're in a fantastic mood. A negative anchor could be having a terrible fight with your spouse. Now every time you see your partner, you instantly feel angry.

Our world is full of anchors

Anchors can operate in any sensory system: sight, sound, touch, taste, or smell. Here is an example of a visual anchor. You see a big truck with advertising on the side of it – maybe a picture of a nice, big ice cream cone. The next thing you know, you're going through the drive-thru to get ice cream. Then the next time you see a big truck with advertising on it, you may think of ice cream again. If you see that same truck over and over, you'll become anchored to ice cream. Wow, you've been programmed and don't even know it!

A sound anchor could be just the way someone says your name. Do you remember when you were young and your mother would use a certain tone of voice when you were doing something wrong? That's an auditory anchor.

Do you remember the story of Ivan Pavlov and his dogs? He conducted experiments in behavioral psychology. Simply put, Pavlov would ring a bell every time food was delivered to the dogs. Eventually, the dogs became so conditioned to the sound of the bell that the sound alone would cause them to salivate, even without the presence of any food

A tactile anchor could be someone touching you in a certain way that gives you this fantastic feeling. Or someone shakes your hand and you get a different feeling. If someone touches you in the same place, over and over when you're in that exact same state, you become anchored to that feeling.

Smell and taste can be particularly powerful anchors. Can you remember a time when you smelled a certain food and it brought up a specific childhood memory? Or how about the taste of your favorite food? That might bring up all kinds of memories. Take notice of the times when you have the urge to go out and impulse eat, and look for the anchors.

Here's an example that involves more than one sense, both sight and sound. An ambulance, like so many other things, is an anchor: a sensory stimulus linked to a specific state. I get chills up my spine every time an ambulance passes. From a purely logical perspective, it's a weird reaction. After all, an ambulance is just a vehicle, with four tires and a motor; it's a form of transportation. There's nothing outrageously exciting about it. But how we interpret its symbolism is another story. Yes, it's a vehicle with wheels, a form of transportation. At the same time, it represents a way to help people in an emergency. When I see an ambulance, I also see a person in need who has the potential to be saved.

Take a moment and think about how you feel when you see an ambulance. You may instantly experience powerful emotions. The sight and sound may link you to a certain experience you had in a hospital, or a health emergency of someone you know.

Companies, slogans and anchors

Especially when it comes to food, there are companies that are masters at anchoring us without us knowing. Advertisers, using television and radio as their medium, anchor us every day, and quite often we have no idea. In essence, we're being hypnotized.

If I were to say, "I'm lovin' it", chances are you'd recognize the McDonald's slogan. Or how about, "We love to see you smile"? McDonald's again. They should anchor with the words, "We love to see you get fat." Do you think we would still be going to McDonald's?

How about the clever fast food chain slogans: "Where's the beef?" or, "It's better here." Wendy's slogans, right? Or what about, "Think outside the bun" or, "Make a run for the border"? You guessed it. Taco Bell.

Some of us knew the answers in a split second. We're anchored to these slogans. They're catchy, sound good, and attempt to trigger you to act and go eat all that unhealthy food. Some of you are so anchored to these slogans and companies that you're in your car right now heading for the drive-thru, just because I mentioned them! If that's you, turn your car around right now because we're going to reprogram you with new, empowering anchors and get rid of those old ones that are holding you back from having the success you so deserve.

Has there ever been a time in your life when you were under stress and you reached for a pile of junk food? You didn't think about it, you just automatically did it. You acted exactly like Pavlov's dogs. I am sure there have been many times when you would've done just about anything to change this behavior.

Unfortunately, the behavior has become unconscious. You go through the drive-thru at the fast food restaurant and barely remember turning in, getting the food, and then eating it. The key to breaking this pattern of acting on your unconscious thoughts is first to become aware of the anchors that are not supporting your goals and eliminate them. Then, replace them with new responses that put you into powerful states that help you achieve your goals.

If you're choosing bad food, you're being steered by negative anchors. They are the source of your impulse eating, binging, overeating, or addiction to junk food. If we create enough positive anchors to healthy foods, you will find yourself naturally inclined to make healthy choices.

The great thing about this technique is that once an anchor is placed, you don't have to think about it to make the associated experience happen. You can create a trigger mechanism that will put you into a powerful state automatically. When you anchor something effectively, it will be at your disposal whenever you need it.

Anchors can either support your success or hold you back from everything you are trying to achieve. Learn to use them to your advantage and watch your success soar.

Change your emotional state in an instant

Once you relate a powerful anchor to a part of your body, you can change your emotional state in a split second. All you have to do is give that anchor a slight squeeze to put yourself in a positive state.

If it sounds too good to be true, think again. I have anchors set all over my body. I touch my earlobe and go into a motivated state. I touch my other ear lobe and I go into a happy state. I touch my knee and I go into a relaxed state.

Once you create these anchors for yourself, at any time you will be to access them to create powerful change. If you can't motivate yourself, anchor motivation. If you want to be happier, anchor happiness. If you want to be more loving, anchor love.

Let me remind you, you don't have a weight problem; you have behavioral and emotional problems. When you're in a great emotional state, it's a lot easier to stay in great shape and choose healthy eating. When I gained 65 pounds of unwanted fat, I was not very happy. But when I got my emotions in check, when I could pull up a great emotion in an instant; my weight and my life started to change.

Let me teach you some ways to anchor yourself and others. The first thing you must do when you set an anchor is to put yourself or the other person into a very specific positive state. If you want to anchor happiness, you must be in a state of happiness. Then, while in that state, you must consistently provide a unique stimulus.

For example, when someone is happy, if you repeatedly squeeze their knee in the exact same place with a unique pressure and attach it to a certain sound, you can create an anchor. Later, you can squeeze their knee in the same spot, make the same sound, and that will instantly put them into a state of happiness.

To have some fun with this anchoring technique, here's a step-by-step exercise to do with a partner to increase your motivation. (You can repeat the exercise for any other state you want to anchor.) Once you anchor this into your nervous system, all you have to do is make one squeeze to instantly go into a motivated state.

1. Ask your partner to remember a time when she was totally motivated, and have her step back into that experience. Make sure she's associated with the event, seeing the experience through her own eyes. Make sure she's feeling the sense of motivation in her body. The greater the emotional intensity, the easier it is to anchor, and the longer-lasting the anchor will be. Also, make sure she stays focused. If she is thinking about two separate things, the anchor will not be as powerful. The stimulus will be linked to two separate things.

2. One of the most important steps is to anchor the experience at its peak state. If you anchor too soon or too late, you will not get the same effect. You will begin to notice changes in her physiology, breathing, facial expressions, and posture. Watch closely for when your partner reaches her peak state. This is when you want to apply the anchor.

3. Place your anchor in a unique place so it gives a clear direction to the brain. For example, if you tried to place an anchor by shaking hands, this would not be very effective because it's not unique and the brain won't get a clear message. Pick your spot and apply pressure. Repeat this several

times while she's in her peak state. Be sure to touch her in the exact same spot each time. You cannot re-trigger an anchor by touching a different place or with a completely different pressure.

4. Release the anchor when the experience begins to fade. If you keep anchoring when the experience is fading, then you will anchor the state of calmness.

5. Test your anchor to see if it has worked. First, have your partner jump up and down and spin around to change her physiology and break the state. Now test the anchor. Simply apply pressure to the exact same place and observe. Does her physiology go into the same state of motivation? If yes, your anchor is effective. If not, you have missed one of the steps, and you must go back and repeat them.

One of the reasons anchoring is so powerful is because it aligns your nervous system with your objective and automatically does what you want. A traditional way to affect change is to think positively, but the problem with this approach is that you have to stop and think!

I get into one of my most powerful states by going into the stance of a warrior. In that stance and that physiology, I have overcome many challenges and accomplished things that I never thought I could do. Going into that stance played a big part in my weight loss. That stance made me feel powerful, like I could achieve anything. When I was in that state, I just knew the weight was coming off; nothing could prevent me from achieving my goals.

What is your why?

You must have a strong enough why to keep you motivated every day to follow through with your weight goals.

_____

_____

_____

_____

Hang your "why" on your wall so you can see it every day. Repeat your why every day until you achieve your goal.

What are three behaviors that are holding you back from achieving your ideal healthy weight?

_____

_____

_____

_____

What are two new behaviors that you can do daily that will help you lose weight for the rest of your life?

_____

_____

_____

_____

Hang these two new behaviors where you can see them and write them in your goal- setting book. Write and re-write your goals daily. This is the fastest way to become successful.

NOTES:

CHAPTER FOUR
Instant Emotional Control

This chapter is about making choices about your state of mind that will help you to achieve your ideal weight, have the healthy body you so deserve, and live a long, fulfilling life. Understanding states is critical to achieving everything you desire. The key to success is to consistently take on an attitude that inspires you to just go out and do it. You don't think about it, you don't talk about it, you just do it. To be able to achieve anything in life, you have to be able get yourself to just go out and do it on a daily basis.

In the Western world, we are taught that mind and body are two separate things. In reality, that's far from the truth. Mind and body inevitably affect each other. So if they affect each other, they must function as a whole. For example, numerous studies have shown that lower back pain can be attributed to emotions around money and the fear of becoming broke. Without a doubt, when it comes to eating, our mind and emotional states are in control of what we do to our bodies.

Think back to a time when you were totally succeeding. I guarantee you were in the most positive states, and those states were pushing you to follow through, to just do it. Can you remember a time when you were sticking to your exercise routine, and every time you weighed yourself you lost a little bit of weight? You achieved one of the most important states; you created a massive amount of momentum. You were on a roll. You would look at the scale and get so excited, and that gave you the momentum to keep going, to keep taking action.

You have also likely had the opposite experience, times when you say to yourself, "I have to go exercise today," but you just can't get yourself motivated. What's the difference? You're the exact same person. You have the exact same skills and talents at your disposal. So why are you "on fire" one day, and the next day you're struggling just to get through the day? One day you stay on your weight loss

69

program, and the next day you're eating everything in sight. The difference is the neurophysiological state you're in.

Let me explain. There are empowering states and disempowering states. Examples of empowering states are confidence, happiness, love, joy, ecstasy, belief, and inner strength, just to name a few. Then there are states that are disempowering, such as frustration, anger, guilt, depression, fear, anxiety, and confusion. These latter types of emotional states leave us feeling helpless. Very often these states lead us into emotional eating, giving up on exercise, mentally beating ourselves up, and so on.

To have success, to achieve your ideal healthy weight and keep it forever, you have to learn how to take action on a consistent basis. And the way you do that is to learn how to put yourself in the most resourceful of states all the time. Yes, there are going to be times when you go into a bad state; that's life. But the real key is to become consciously aware of when you go into negative states, and be able to pull yourself out of that state in a matter of seconds. Most of the time, we put on weight because we get into negative states and we stay in those states for long periods of time, day in and day out, month after month, or for some of us, year after year.

If you can get control of your emotional states throughout the day, very soon, not only will you win the war on weight loss, but you will also prevent stress and disease from entering your body. It's very hard to allow stress and disease to impact the body when you're brimming with happiness and vitality, full of energy, and striving to have the body you so deserve. Once you get control of your emotional states on a daily basis, your life will completely change.

Think about why people overeat. It's often to soothe uncomfortable emotions. Food can take the focus off of anger, resentment, fear, anxiety, and a host of other emotions we'd sometimes rather not feel.

When he feels bad, my friend, Jim, loves to binge on junk food. At first, he gets good feelings from the food. For a short period of time serotonin is produced, and it begins to turn off his appetite and turn on his good mood, giving him instant gratification. Soon, however, the emotion of guilt creeps up on him and he enters into a state that disempowers him. And the cycle continues. If Jim changed his state, he could change his behavior.

How you respond to other people's states is just as important as managing your own. For example, if your friend eats a bunch of junk food, ends up in a state of guilt, and lashes out at you, instead of getting angry at that person, you could choose to come from a place of compassion. You know that's not who they really are; it's just the state they're in at that time.

Why choose to put yourself into a disempowering state to play their game? Once you enter that state, you too are at risk of choosing to emotionally eat, losing your motivation to exercise, and giving up on your goals. If you choose to consistently put yourself into negative states, you have a good chance of introducing disease into your body. Do not get caught up in this trap! Watch how other people's states are affecting your own.

What exactly is a "state", and why does it matter?

State control is one of the most important things you will ever learn. It will help you achieve your ideal healthy weight and maintain it for good. State control equals weight control. Just think how exciting it's going to be when you're able to snap your fingers and put yourself into a state of high energy: you're excited for life, you're sure of success, your mind is alive. My goal is to teach you how to literally snap your fingers and instantly go into these great frames of mind that will consistently give you fantastic feelings and motivate you to take action. You are going to learn how to control your states to make them work for you.

So what is a "state"? It's the sum of the millions of neurological processes happening within you which defines what you're experiencing at any given moment. There are two main considerations to understanding what puts you into empowering or disempowering states. First we'll discuss internal representations; then we'll explore physiology. When you link these two together – internal representations + physiology — they produce a state, and that state drives behavior.

Internal representations include the pictures and thoughts you create in your mind (content) and how you create them (process). Most of our internal representations have become habitual patterns that we learned in our earliest years from other people. They make up our beliefs, attitudes, values, and interpretations. Now don't get scared and think you're stuck in the model your parents have provided for you. You can change it. What really matters now is how you represent things to yourself. Throughout this chapter, I am going to teach you to represent things to yourself in a way that will empower you instead of placing limitations on you. It's your choice how you want to represent things. How you think is connected to your nervous system, so what I am going to do is give you a brand new way to run your nervous system so you can produce positive results.

If you spend the majority of your days in an uplifted, positive emotional state, you're not going to turn to food to get a quick hit of good feelings. Moreover, when you spend most of your days in uplifted emotional states, it's a lot easier to get yourself to exercise day in and day out. As a result, you'll live a longer, healthier life.

What does physiology mean? Your physiology includes numerous elements: muscle tension, food intake, breathing rate, posture, and overall level of biochemical functions.

These bodily functions greatly affect your state. In a state of happiness, you will be walking around, smiling and glowing, your body will be upright, and you will be full of life. So your internal representations (what and how you picture things and talk to yourself), combined with your physiology (how you hold your body, how you breathe, your facial expressions), create your state. This state then governs your behavior.

I hope you understand why this is one of the most important things you will ever learn. Think about when you feel physically vibrant and alive. Don't you perceive the world differently from when you're overweight and out of shape? People who achieve their goals in life are people who have learned to tap into their most resourceful states. The amount of time you spend in positive, uplifted states each day is going to determine your overall success.

Everything we want in life is simply the desire for a state. Actually, there is only one thing in the whole world that each one of us wants, and that is some kind of positive state. We only differ in the methods we use to achieve it. Do you want to eat that chocolate cake? That cake will put you in a state by evoking a feeling or emotion. But it's not the junk food you really want, it's the state the junk food will provide for you.

Is it really a relationship you want? No, you want the state that relationship will put you in. Relationships are supposed to give us good feelings, like love, happiness, excitement, and so on. But just think if you could consistently give yourself those good feelings and not have to turn to food or to somebody else to achieve this. Now I am not saying you must live a solitary existence. What I am saying is that when you know how to control your own state, you don't need to turn to food, drugs, alcohol, cigarettes, or other people for those good feelings. You can rely on your own personal power.

Control your state, control your life

There's only one way to have lifelong success, and that's to become the master over your states and over yourself. Let me give you an example of how people put themselves into certain states. Let's say you just finished making a nice, healthy meal for your spouse. It's a Friday night and he is over an hour late coming home from work. You're getting impatient. You start to create pictures of your spouse in your head. He is having an affair; he must be out with that co-worker. You think, "I knew he liked her." The pictures and the self-talk you are flooding your mind with are going to create your state, and that state is not happiness, its anger. When he finally walks through the door, you're in a state of anger, and you say in an accusatory tone, "Where were you?" He looks puzzled. Then, reaching from behind his back, he hands you a dozen roses and says, "Trying to find you flowers, honey." You now have an instant state change, perhaps to one of embarrassment or of loving feelings towards him, but in return, you may have put him into a bad state.

What would have happened if you were thinking that he was late because he loves you and he may be trying to do something nice for you, like buying you flowers? The pictures and your self-talk would have created a completely different outcome when he walked through the door. Your state would have been inviting and happy. Your behavior would have reflected this. "Oh, honey, I am so happy you're home. How come you're late?" And in responding to you, his state would've remained positive. The truth is, most of us think the worst first, and this directs our state and how we act toward everyone around us.

We need to change our internal representations and physiology so they work together. Once the two are in sync, difficult tasks become effortless. When you tackle tough challenges, such as exercise or healthy eating, positive representations put your physiology into a positive state. And this state produces the behavior you will engage in.

To control and direct our behavior, we must control and direct our states.

Take, for example, the emotional state of stress. In times of stress, few things can be as powerfully comforting or rewarding as food. This is because we have not developed effective coping strategies. If you provide a person with the right strategy, and they have a strong enough belief system, their coping response to stress will completely change.

We have lots of anchors in us that create our states, but most of us do not realize that they are at our disposal. These anchors start pinning us to states when we are young. Maybe your parents rewarded you with sweets, soothed your hurt with an ice cream cone, or took you to McDonald's to celebrate your success. The vast majority of us have developed emotional attachments to food because we were programmed this way. People eat to celebrate, to deal with stress, to change their state, to feel better about themselves, and so on.

In neuro-linguistic programming (NLP), you learn a very important concept: the map is not the territory. What this means is that how we represent things to ourselves is just an interpretation of the event. Most of us want to believe that our perception is the only possibility, and that it's one hundred percent right. But that's just your own map of the territory. If you don't change your map, I can promise you that your life will remain stuck exactly where it is right now. As Einstein famously said, "No problem can be solved from the same level of consciousness that created it." Keep doing the same things, and you will keep getting the same results.

Choose positive representations

There is no objective reality; our perception of the world

comes from our own unique perspective. We filter the information that comes to us through our own system of beliefs, values, and attitudes. Even the highest achievers in the world can think of things that aren't working, and put themselves into emotional states of guilt, frustration, depression, fear, and helplessness. But every high achiever has developed the skill to shift out of that state in a matter of seconds. You have the choice to focus on things that work in your life rather than focus on things that don't work. If you see yourself as healthy, fit, thin, and enjoying exercise, you're going to put yourself into a motivated state. If you see yourself huffing and puffing, and hating exercise, you're going to put yourself into an unmotivated state. So why not choose representations that put you in empowering states instead of disempowering states?

No matter how bad a situation in your life gets, you can choose to represent it in a way that empowers you. This is really taking control of your emotions, your mind, and your life. The people who achieve their ideal healthy weight, the ones who enjoy a great, healthy body, are the ones who can gain access to their most resourceful states on a consistent basis.

A woman I know named Sarah understands the power of states. Five years ago, just after she graduated, Sarah decided to take her own life. Lying across some railroad tracks, she could hear the train coming closer and closer, until it ran right over her. Sarah's body was split in two, the bottom half completely severed from the upper half. She lay screaming in pain. You would think she would have died, but she didn't.

Sarah survived. She lives today without the lower half of her body. She had to decide how to go on living, and the only way was to represent the event in a way that would put her into a positive state. Despite being cut in half, Sarah found a way to do this. Now she speaks about her experience around the world, and helps people live better lives. Sarah could have just given up, but she chose instead to change the pictures in her head and how she talked to herself.

Nothing is inherently good or bad. We choose how we represent things to ourselves. We can represent things in a way that lifts us up or that tears us down. Just like Sarah, who decided to represent things to herself in a positive, uplifting way, we all have that choice.

In my seminars, I take a long, sharp pin and stick it into a board so the sharp end is sticking up. I then get my seminar attendees to smash their hands onto the pin with the intention of crushing it flat. If they hesitate or doubt themselves, the pin will go right through their hand. So they have to represent the event to themselves in an empowering light. They have to come from a place of belief that they can do it, putting themselves in the most powerful state so they can follow through and succeed. Just like life.

The pin exercise teaches people how to change their states and their behaviors in a way that gets them motivated to take action, in spite of fear and doubt. It gets them to break old patterns and limitations. The only way people can do this exercise is if they change their physiology and their internal representations of what they can and cannot do. Their old state would have prohibited them from following through, but their new state enables them to do what previously seemed impossible.

Think about this scenario. If I say to you, "Let's go for a day's hike up a mountain," what does this stimulate in your brain? What happens is, when I say that statement your brain produces a representation. If you picture yourself walking up the mountain, having a great day getting in shape; if you say to yourself, "I can do this"; and if you position your body as if you were totally confident, the neurological signals that you will produce will put you into a state in which you believe you can hike up the mountain. However, if you picture yourself barely making it up the mountain, sweating, hating it, seeing yourself only half way up the mountain and stopping to throw up, you're not going to put yourself into a state that encourages you to follow through.

It's exactly the same thing with your life. If you represent things to yourself as if they're not going to work, you're right, they won't. I can assure you of that. If you form representations of yourself achieving your weight goals, achieving your life goals, then you will put yourself into those states that will produce the results that you want to achieve.

Can you see how important it is to make the right internal representations in your mind? Your brain can stop you from succeeding or guide you to all the success you have ever dreamed of. Donald Trump, Oprah Winfrey, and people who successfully keep their weight off forever make representations of the world as a place where they can achieve any result they truly desire. The right representations determine your state, your state determines your behavior, and your behavior determines your results.

Your physiology and success

Now let's talk about how important it is to be able to use your physiology in the right way to achieve massive success. Physiology is the most powerful tool you have for instantly changing your state and producing amazing results. Once you learn how to change your physiology, you can automatically put yourself into states of confidence and motivation. It's very easy to get yourself to take action when your physiology is doing the work for you.

You hear me talk a lot about how the key to success is taking action. And the way you get yourself to take action is to act as if you're already there. Act as if you were already in great shape. Act as if you have all the resources at your disposal to succeed. Act as if you were totally energized. Act as if you were already thin. Act as if your body was exactly how you wanted it to be. Once you put your physiology into a state of acting "as if", it becomes a very powerful tool for change.

In my seminars, I am constantly getting people into their most powerful physiology. I have them do some of the craziest things. Not because I like to see people dance around like fools, or yell at the top of their lungs while pumping their fists in the air, but because when you get them into their most powerful physiology, people can produce the most amazing results, results that will change their lives. Remember, your physiology is your posture, your breathing pattern, your tonal fluctuations, your muscle tension. When you change your physiology, you automatically change your internal representations, which in turn change your state.

Mind and body work together

So, you see, it works both ways. Mind and body inevitably affect each other. In Western culture, we're told mind and body are separate, but they're not; they're two parts of a whole. Think about a time when you have had pain in your body. I guarantee you perceived the world differently than when you were pain-free. Is that not convincing enough evidence that mind and body are one?

Your physiology is the master key to emotional change. Sit up straight right now — fast, sit up! Put a big smile on your face. I guarantee your emotional state just changed dramatically. It's hard to maintain a negative emotional state when your physiology reflects an uplifting, confident manner. This technique can be used when you feel you can't succeed at something. By changing how you're standing, how you're breathing, and the tone of voice you are using, you can enter into states that will help you follow through and achieve the things you're after.

Take exercise, for example. The fact is, one of the major reasons people are overweight and out of shape is that they have trouble getting themselves to exercise on a consistent basis. Let's say you're on the treadmill, and you keep saying to yourself that you're so tired you just can't go on. This language will put your physiology into a state that will reflect those thoughts. Before long, you're tired, your posture is slumped, and you're breathing heavily. Soon, you're sitting on the floor and can't go on.

If instead you were to say things to yourself like, "I love exercising. I am healthy and fit. I can do this," you would actually start to put yourself into a state of enjoying exercise. Even if you detest exercise, if you condition your nervous system by changing your physiology, eventually you will start to love it.

Here's another example of mind and body working together. Have you heard of laughing yoga? I was teaching a seminar once, and one of the other presenters was a laughing yoga instructor, so he had everyone following these laughing yoga exercises. I have to admit, at first I thought this was the most ridiculous thing I had ever seen, but I decided to go along with it. It was a new experience, and the more I did this laughing yoga, the better the state I found myself in. When we smile and laugh, we set off a biochemical reaction that makes us feel good. The problem is that, as adults, we laugh an average of only seven times per day. Kids laugh about seventy-seven times per day!

Model congruency

Congruency is critical to succeeding with your weight, health, and life goals. What I mean by congruency is creating a sense of internal and external harmony; you have to walk your talk. Think about this. If you're thinking about how you're going to achieve your ideal healthy weight, and you're repeating positive messages, but your tone and your body language are weak, you are in a state of incongruence. And incongruence can literally sabotage all the success you want in your life.

If you want to be the best you can possibly be in everything you do, if you want to be able to stick with your weight loss goals, your health goals, and stay motivated, it is crucial that you become congruent. Once you master congruency, you will produce outstanding results in every area of your life. You really only have to accomplish the skill of congruence in one area of your life and it will affect all other areas of your life.

Successful people have mastered congruency, so model them. Pick three people you know who are extremely congruent, and mirror exactly what they do. How do they hold their bodies? How do they sit? How do they stand? How do they move? What are their facial expressions like? What type of gestures do they make? How is their physiology different from yours?

Take a moment and stand exactly the way one of these people would stand. Mimic one of their facial expressions and gestures. Now notice how different you feel. By mirroring their physiology, you will start to send signals to your brain to produce the results you're after.

You've probably heard the saying, "You become like the people you surround yourself with." If you hang around with people who are depressed, it's easy to start to mirror their physiology. In fact, you start doing this unconsciously, and soon you're wondering why you're in a state of depression.

If you don't have a lot of people around you to model, find a DVD of anybody you would like to mirror – Martin Luther King Jr., a dynamic motivational speaker – and do exactly what you see on the DVD. Breathe like they breathe. Use the same tonality. Move the way they move. You will start to activate the same parts of the brain they do. Once you understand how to do this, and after you have done it a few times, you can start to tap into parts of your brain that will free you from the struggle you have had with weight for so many years.

You now have ways to change your state without having to turn to destructive things like food, alcohol, drugs, and the many things we turn to that harm our bodies and our health. By breathing differently, moving your body differently, having different facial expressions, you create new patterns that will give you the same result as food, drugs, alcohol, smoking, and other destructive habits. You will change your state by changing your physiology in healthy ways.

State change exercise

Let's do an exercise that will teach you how to get into an uplifting emotional state at any time. Most of us are a lot better at putting ourselves into states like frustration, stress, depression, anger, guilt, or feeling overwhelmed, just to name a few. Once you learn how to put yourself into empowering states on a consistent basis, your life will completely change. Being in a positive emotional state will help you take action, follow through, and give you the extra drive you need to succeed.

Here is what I want you to do. Think of a dream that you would just love to achieve, something that gets you really excited. I want you to think of this dream as achievable; no matter what, you can make this thing happen. Stay focused on this dream that gets you emotionally charged up, as if you could not live without it.

Now I want you to sit the way you would be sitting if you were just wishing this dream would happen, as opposed to feeling absolutely certain you will achieve it. How would you hold your body? Say to yourself, "I wish this would happen." Put the expression on your face that matches your state of just wishing. Experience that state you're putting yourself in right now. Really feel those feelings. Now stand up, and stand like you're just wishing that this dream would happen. Make a gesture as you repeat your dream again. "I wish I could achieve my health goals." "I wish I could live a long, healthy life." "I wish I could make it to the gym five days per week." I wish I were happier." "I wish I had a good spouse." "I wish I had a new spouse."

Say the words to yourself once more, as if you were just wishing your dream would happen, and take a close look at your physiology. Notice how you were breathing. Was it short and fast, or long and slow? Notice your tone. Was it quiet or loud, varied or monotone? Did you talk fast or slow? What happened with your body? Did you rock back and forth? Did you stand to one side? Were your shoulders slumped or pulled back? Was your head up, looking down, or turned to the side? Was there tension in your body? Notice how you made your gesture. Was it slow and careless, or fast and precise?

Now repeat your dream again in this state of just wishing, and pay close attention to your internal representations. It's important to understand how you create these states that hold you back. What did you picture in your head as you were in this state of wishing? Did you picture exercise being hard, or you fighting with someone? Become consciously aware of the kind of pictures you create in your head to get yourself into this state. Did you see yourself succeeding, or did you see yourself failing? Was the picture in your head near or far, bright or dim, big or small? Were you associated or dissociated? Associated means you are seeing the event through your own eyes. Dissociated means you are floating above yourself, and seeing the event from above. Did you feel "blah"? Or did you feel nothing at all?

I'll bet your speech slowed down, your movements slowed, and you may have rocked back and forth. Your breathing probably became shallow; the pictures in your head became dark, distorted and dim; and you saw things not working out. You may have stood to one side. This is what most of us do when we get ourselves into these disempowering states.

State of total confidence

Now put yourself into a state of total confidence. Create a picture in your head of total confidence. Stand the way you would stand if you were totally confident. Breathe the way you would breathe. Create the expression on your face and make a gesture as if you were totally confident. What would you be saying to yourself? What is your tonality like? How would you hold your head? Where is the energy in your body? Go right into that state. Experience it right now.

This is the state you want to be able to access at any time to have great success. Feel that state; be in that state; enjoy that state. Say these words to yourself with conviction: "I'm going to find or make a way because I just know I can. I'm going to get the weight off and keep it off forever this time." Put that determined look on your face as if you're going to find a way no matter what obstacles confront you. No matter what it takes, you're just going to make it happen. Nothing is going to stop you. Then add to that a feeling of excitement. You feel confident, and it excites you to know that you're going to make it happen. You're excited for the new body you're going to create. Even if it seems impossible, you will find a way and you will get there.

I want you to do whatever it takes right now, even if you think it is impossible, to double your confidence in your ability to create a new body. Now doesn't this state feel a lot different than when you were just wishing for something to happen? What would your life be like if you could access this state at any time? Do you think that you may be more motivated to achieve your goals? Of course! Now let's go back and look at what you did to get yourself totally confident.

Notice your posture. Were your shoulders pulled back? How were your feet placed? Were they firmly on the ground? Did you lean forward? What did you picture in your mind? Notice if the pictures were near, big, and bright. Could you see things working out for you? What did you say to yourself? What tone did you use? Was your speech fast or slow? Was it loud or soft? What were your facial expressions like? How about your gestures? Were they different from when you were just wishing? Were they strong with the conviction that you were going to succeed?

Now when you're in this strong state of confidence, do you think you can lose all the weight? Yes! When you're in this state, if your boss walks up to you and says, "You're fired!" what would you say? "Fantastic! I was ready for bigger things anyway." If someone were mean to you when you're in this state, what would you say next? What could you do in this state? Anything! You can achieve anything because you just find or make a way. You don't even know what the word failure means. You just keeping going and going and going until you achieve the thing you want. If someone says to you "You're overweight!" when you are in this state, you will say, "Yes, thanks. Watch me get in great shape. Now get out of my way!" This is all it takes for you to become extremely successful in anything that you do, and that is to understand how to put yourself into a powerful state. This is what is really going to get you to keep exercising day in and day out. This sense of power is what gives you the motivation. It goes a lot deeper than just saying that you are motivated. By finding the power to be motivated, you can produce lasting change in your weight and your life.

Once you discover the strategies that will change your thought processes, you no longer have outside forces controlling you. You will no longer give the key to your brain away, as you do the key to your house. And that's exactly what you're doing here, finding out how to operate your brain. Now you should be convinced that all you have to do is make some small changes in your state, and you can completely change how you see things. The behavior you are engaging in has a powerful ability to take you out of any kind of negative emotion you're in at the time. When you're in a good emotional state, you can produce outstanding results in anything. State control really does equal weight control. In fact, state control equals life control. Remember how easy the process is. Control the internal representations running in your head and change your physiology and, "voila!" you have a change of state.

Rewiring the brain

I have a client who was having a lot of trouble trying to change her state. Whenever she was alone, she would eat everything in sight, whatever she could get her hands on. It was only when she was by herself that she would start to binge. After a modest meal, she would wait for guests to leave her place, then she would eat everything in the cupboard. I mean, everything, until there was hardly anything left; until she made herself sick. It became a very deeply rooted anchor for her. Every time she started to binge, she held her body in a certain way, her head was lowered, and her internal dialogue reflected a negative tone and disempowering words. She became used to engaging in this destructive behavior to the point where it would not feel normal if she did not conduct herself this way. She had lost control of herself, and her self-esteem was at an all-time low.

The way she finally got control over herself was to change her focus. She had been focusing on wanting to binge when nobody was around. By figuring out how she was training her brain for disaster, we were able to fix the problem. We helped her change her focus and her physiology, and rewire her brain. To this day, she has not once gone back to her old pattern, and enjoys a very healthy lifestyle.

Master your emotions

The key to mastering your emotions is to become consciously aware of when negative emotions surface, and learn to redirect yourself. Here's what I want you to do for the next two to five days.

The first step is to record and appreciate your emotions. It's very important to record your negative emotions when they arise. Have a journal handy specifically for this task. When you notice a negative emotion emerging, write down what brought it on, and then how you dealt with it. Once you recognize the negative emotion, learn to appreciate it for what it may teach you.

The second step is to analyze the emotion. How is the emotion directing you? Is it telling you to look at the situation from a different perspective? What direction are you going in, and should you be changing direction?

Step three is to redirect. In order to change an emotion and the direction you are taking, ask yourself the right questions. What emotion do I really want to feel? What would I have to change in order to feel that now? What action will I take to change my state right now? What positives can I take from this?

Step four is to get confident. Think back to other difficult situations that challenged you, and how you worked through them. This time you even have more tools to use.

Follow this formula and you will start to produce positive emotional states on a consistent basis, and that's really the path to success. So for the next two to five days, really work on noticing when your negative emotions come up, and follow the steps I have just laid out for you. Then, watch your life change.

Do something new

We've talked a lot about the power of changing your state, and several ways to do this. Here's one more tool you can use: do something new. Most of us do the same things over and over, and eventually, they become boring. The frontal lobe, the most powerful part of your brain, thrives on newness. So expand your options, and you will find it that much easier to access positive states.

Make a list of all the things that make you feel great. Here are some examples. Sing your favorite song. Take ten deep breaths. Name twenty-five things you are grateful for. Watch an inspirational movie. Call someone and tell them you love them. Exercise. Pump your fist in the air and shout, "I am awesome!" ten times. Meditate. Grab your favorite book. There are literally thousands of ways to change your state so you produce positive emotions. Use this list daily when you need to quickly change your state.

CHAPTER FIVE
Learn What Science Has Taught Us About The Frontal Lobe Of The Brain And Weight Loss

The right questions combined with mental repetition will fully activate the frontal lobe.

In your quest to achieve success in life, including your weight and health, this is probably the best hidden secret that you will ever learn. It is a subject that you have probably heard very little about. People like Oprah, Will Smith, Martin Luther King Jr., Gandhi, Madonna, and Mother Theresa have all learned to tap into this resource at a deep level. We often think that these people are endowed with brain structures that are different from ours. Why do so few people achieve the same level of success as their heroes? It's not that our heroes are any smarter or better than the rest of us. They have just learned to do one thing critical for success, and that one thing is something that you can also learn to do.

So what is this thing that's going to help you think like the great leaders of the world? All right, here it is: This great resource used by the most successful people in history is the part of your brain called the frontal lobe.

I'm thrilled to teach you this secret. Simply by tapping into the frontal lobe, we're going to change all those old patterns and habits that have been keeping your goals and success at bay. Once you start to actively engage this part of your brain on a daily basis, your weight will change, your life will change, and you will start to achieve greatness at whatever you set your mind to. You will be thinking from the same mindset employed by the doers of this world.

What is the frontal lobe?

So what on earth is the frontal lobe, and what does it have to do with achieving your ideal, healthy weight? Rather than go into too many technical terms and bore you, let me summarize. The frontal lobe sits at the front and center of the brain. It is the largest of the four lobes, and is the most highly developed part of the human nervous system. The frontal lobe is the emotional control center of the brain.

What you are about to learn shakes up the traditional approach to changing behaviors. You've probably heard it before: your thoughts become feelings, your feelings become actions, and your actions become results. So it would look like this: Thoughts = feelings = actions = results. But the brain simply does not work like that. What happens is you have a thought that produces a feeling, and then the feeling loops back to the thought. So it goes like this. Thoughts = feelings = thoughts = feelings = thoughts. Thinking, feeling; feeling, thinking; thinking, feeling. And so the vicious cycle goes on. We need to learn to break this cycle so we can move forward to taking action, and get the results we're after. If we choose to break this cycle, we automatically tap into the power of the frontal lobe.

The Gatekeeper

It wasn't too long ago when I asked one of my multi-millionaire mentors, "What do you think is the secret to making over 100 million dollars?" His response was, "Well, Shane, in every industry, every venture that I went into, I found the gatekeeper, the person who could open the door for me. I did whatever it took to get to the person who had that key."

If I were to say to you right now, "I have access to your gatekeeper, the person that can open all the doors to your dreams, whatever career you're in, whatever stage of life you're at," would you take the key or would you walk away? Of course you would take it. It's like winning the lottery. The frontal lobe functions as a gatekeeper to manage information, and determine whether to shut it out, put it aside and attend to it later, or put it front and center. You have the gatekeeper at your disposal right now.

The frontal lobe is the gatekeeper. Once we get through the gates, we can take efficient and effective action to produce the results we're after. Can you remember a time when you just could not get yourself motivated to go exercise? The gates were closed. You start thinking thoughts like how bad it was going to be; how much work it would be; how hard it is; and how you might sweat. The more you started thinking, the more you started to produce a feeling of not wanting to follow through. That feeling would go back to a thought; for example, of how exercise is hard, and that thought would then reinforce your lack of motivation. These thoughts create barriers that keep you from moving to the action stage. In fact, it is pretty much impossible if the gates are closed. You end up with an outcome that you were trying to prevent: gaining more weight. Very few of us end up seeing the results we want because we're stuck in the thinking-and-feeling, feeling-and-thinking cycle.

The frontal lobe is the part of the brain that provides us with the power to become unstuck, to break out of unhealthy patterns. It is here that we can choose between good and bad (do not eat the whole cake, versus eat the whole cake). And it is here that we associate emotions with memories (the last time I ate the whole chocolate cake, I became moody and depressed following the sugar high.) And, fortunately, it is here that we can break negative cycles.

If the frontal lobe is such an important piece of the puzzle for us to create success in our lives, why then do so few of us utilize it to achieve our full potential? The reason is that most of us become addicted to our emotions. In a very real sense, we have become caught in the trap of doing the same things over and over again. Our brains become accustomed to our daily routines, which require little or no thought. We start to crave those routines, and we don't want to experience new things that are unfamiliar to us. If someone throws us off our routine, we're completely lost.

We start to live our lives in a catatonic state. We become lazy, unmotivated, and uninspired. We have difficulty focusing in on one single task at hand. When we start a project, or go on a new diet or a new exercise program, or read a new book, we never seem to follow through with it. We become good starters but not good finishers. The people who get rewards in life are the ones who can finish.

Be honest; does any of this sound like you? Don't be in denial; the first step is to become aware and take full responsibility. This is the only way you can make a change in your life. So don't sell yourself short.

Emotionally impulsive behavior

The latest scientific brain research shows that the less you use your frontal lobe, the greater chance you have of responding with impulsive, overly emotional behavior. Our emotions are what lead us to impulse eating, and farther away from success in every area of our life. When our frontal lobe is fully engaged, we have the power to have more control over our emotional impulse behaviors. The sooner you start to tap into this resource called the frontal lobe, the sooner you can be on the road to becoming the person you would like to be.

Our personalities are dominated by the cycle of neurological and chemical responses that occur in the body. Most of these responses are memories of the past, which dictate the choices we make and the reactions we set in motion. In essence, we become addicted to these repetitive chemical reactions that keep us living in survival mode. If we can start thinking beyond how we feel, and our emotional responses, then we can start to move beyond living in survival mode, and change the repetitive chemical reactions in our body.

Once I started to learn about the frontal lobe and really put it into action, my life started to completely change. I started to think differently, act differently, and make better choices. I call the frontal lobe a gift we have all been given. The problem is most of us never unwrap this great gift. It sits there in the wrapping paper for years and years, often never utilized to its fullest potential. When you're given a Christmas or birthday present, you don't just sit there and stare at it, or say, "I am going to wait two years to open this." No, you're so excited that you just want to tear the paper open. This is how you should look at the frontal lobe. You have been given a gift, and you are now going to unwrap this gift and learn how to use it to its full potential. Like a video game, once you get really good at it and master it, the game becomes easy. The same process of mastery applies to your frontal lobe. Once you get really good at using the frontal lobe to your advantage, you will start to master your life. It's time for you to step up and unwrap this great gift called the frontal lobe.

If we were to take away our frontal lobe, we would be similar to every other species. A cat's frontal lobe makes up 3.5% of its higher brain anatomy; a dog has a little more than a cat, at 7%; and a chimpanzee, 11 to 17%. In humans, the frontal lobe makes up 30 to 40% of the higher brain anatomy. We have unparalleled potential to use the frontal lobe and control it. What is the sense in not utilizing this gift, and acting like every other species?

Gain mastery over the frontal lobe

Right now, I'll bet you're not aware of your surroundings, the noises that are going on around you, the breath you are taking in and out, the feelings you are feeling in your body, the taste in your mouth, the smells in the air, the pain in your leg, the smile on your face. All you may be focused on are the words that you are reading right now. That's your frontal lobe at work. It centers all of your attention. You may have just turned the page in this book or looked at the clock across the room, scratched your leg, looked out the window, or performed any of a thousand different actions you may make while reading this book.

The frontal lobe is responsible for all the conscious choices and actions you make in a day. Think of it as a conductor on a train. The conductor makes all the decisions to guide the train down the track to get to the final destination. Your frontal lobe has access to all other parts of the brain; like the conductor of the train, the frontal lobe has complete control over the rest of the brain and how it operates. No other part of the brain has the capability to operate at such a high level. If we are ever going to be able to create a change in our behavior, and think rather than just feel, we need to become familiar with the frontal lobe and how it works.

The frontal lobe has the privilege of being the captain of the ship. And it loves to learn new things. So keep learning! The frontal lobe likes to stay focused on what's new and exciting. When a skill is new, fun, and exciting, the frontal lobe is like a kid at Christmas. It unwraps what's new for you and is inspired to try it out. Now, after a few repetitions, when all the newness and excitement is gone, the frontal lobe passes the work to other parts of the brain. This is the privilege it gets for being the captain of the ship. The work is now passed down to the grunts so they can do the mundane, routine work.

The frontal lobe also keeps us focused on what's important. Do you remember a time when you had the ability to stay determinedly focused, to stick with your health and fitness goals? This is because the frontal lobe cools off other neural signals, so that you do not become distracted by information that takes you away from your goals. It's like tuning into the radio station you choose to listen to. It removes the static of fuzzy thinking, allowing you to be more creative, and to examine, analyze, and focus on what you really want.

If we don't learn to direct the frontal lobe, our daily thoughts become concerned with the survival of our body, and if we're just concerned with survival, then how can we create a compelling future? How can we create a healthy lifestyle? How can we create our dreams? We can't, because we're so preoccupied with just getting by.

Our attention, what we focus on, can be our greatest gift or our greatest downfall. We can see into the future or we can anchor ourselves to our past. It's your choice whether you're going to make the decision to start working with this incredible resource. I can't do it for you. I can provide you with the tools. I can lead you to the gatekeeper. But I can't take the action for you; you must follow through. I am going to ask you to make a commitment to work with your frontal lobe every day.

Model Buddhist monks

Many of us have heard of how Buddhist monks can meditate for hours, even days, with extremely focused concentration. This level of control is something we would all love to have, and something that we all can have. There was an experiment conducted on the frontal lobe of Buddhist monks. The monks were asked to hold the thought of compassion. They showed levels of one kind of electrical brain impulses, called gamma waves, that were higher than researchers had ever seen. In one Buddhist monk, the left frontal region was enhanced so much that the researchers concluded he must be the happiest man alive. The happiest man alive! I truly believe that with some work learning to control our emotions through our frontal lobe, we can all achieve that level of success. Yes, we can all be extremely happy. The Buddhist monks did this by learning to quiet the other parts of the brain so they could hold one single thought in their minds.

We can train the brain for maximum results so it functions at a higher level than we could ever possibly imagine. Just like the Buddhist monk who became quite possibly the happiest man in the world, when you learn to control your frontal lobe, you can stay focused on following through with your exercise, you can hold the picture of the body you want in your brain until you get there, you can start to run your brain at an entirely different level.

Countless in-shape individuals have learned to utilize the frontal lobe. The more attentive we become, the higher the level the frontal lobe operates at. Have you ever noticed that when you decide to overeat, you feel controlled by the idea of eating? Let's say you have a thought in your head about going through the drive-thru at McDonald's, and you just know you should not act on that thought, but you can't seem to control yourself. When we gain control of our frontal lobe, we can start to think differently instead of act on those thoughts that are going to leave us with unwanted consequences.

Sometimes teenagers act on certain impulses without really thinking. This is because their frontal lobe is still not fully developed. Similarly, grown-ups sometimes act in the same way as teenagers because they're not actively using their frontal lobe. I am going to show you how to use the frontal lobe to have the impulse control of a disciplined adult, a level of impulse control that reflects your maturity and intelligence. Those impulses to just go out and act can become a thing of the past.

There was a time in my life when I wondered why I couldn't get myself to follow through on things. When I was overweight, I would say, "Tomorrow I am going to the gym." Then tomorrow would come and I would say the exact same thing again. I would find myself going for ice cream after dinner rather than going for a good, revitalizing walk. Why could I not get myself to follow through? I had to find the answer so I could create a change in my life.

How come when we say, "I am going to stop drinking pop," we don't follow through with what we say? "I am going to be more patient with my spouse." "I am going to help a charity." "I am going to read a book a month." We don't follow through on any of the promises that we make to ourselves. How come we don't take action on things that could greatly improve our lives?

First among our excuses, we just don't feel like it. We start running on automatic pilot – our days, weeks, months, and years start to become exactly the same. We start to respond to that constant chatter in our head every day, and so we end up making that our reality. Whatever the constant chatter is telling us, we follow. The frontal lobe decides to go completely to sleep, and we start responding solely to our feelings. You might say, "I had a hard day at work. I am so tired and drained. I deserve an ice cream to make me feel better." You're responding to your feelings.

Activate your frontal lobe and I guarantee that you will think before you react to those feelings. You will quiet the inner chatter that is trying so hard to talk you out of our dreams and aspirations, your goal to have a long, healthy life, with a fantastic, fit body. The frontal lobe is not only the gatekeeper, but it also acts like your personal secretary. It gives you a plan of action, organizes your thinking, looks at situations with a clear focus, helps you follow through on your plan, guides you to take the right action, and steers you away from the wrong ones based on what you define as your purpose.

Immediate gratification vs. long-term success

Imagine this scenario. It's 11:00 a.m. on Sunday morning and you are set to go out for a workout. You have been doing extremely well. You have stayed on your program for the last two weeks, and you really feel like you're going to do it this time. You're going to achieve your ideal, healthy weight, and keep the excess pounds off. After you do your workout, you meet your friend for lunch and order a nice, healthy salad. Your frontal lobe is precisely clear on what you have to keep doing to ensure your future success.

Now let's look at this scenario. On your way to the gym, you see that your favorite store has a sidewalk sale on, and outside the store you see one of your best friends. On the rack outside, you spot an outfit you have wanted for months. The colors, the design, and the 75% off sign get you so excited that you forget your initial purpose. Your feelings start to override what you really want to accomplish in the end – that ideal, healthy, in-shape body. You pull into the parking lot, yelling out the window to your friend. You start to shop and chat. You're having a great time, and hours have passed. You're getting hungry and no longer feel like going to the gym. Instead you go for lunch with your friend, and you start beating yourself up inside for not following through with going to the gym. So you order comfort food: a big plate of pasta.

If you choose the second option, this is what happens. When you see your best friend at the store, the outfit hanging on the rack, and the 75% off sign, the external stimuli are so distracting that you completely lose your focus. Your mind wanders to other stimuli; what else is going on around the store? Your brain's distraction mechanism stops you from restraining your mind. The focus of your original plan, going to the gym, is completely lost. The frontal lobe's new intention becomes shopping. Your behavior is now no longer matched to your purpose of having your ideal, healthy body. You start to succumb to immediate gratification instead of long-term success. How many of us do this in our lives on a consistent basis?

I think each and every one of us is guilty of this. But the cool thing is we can learn to change it. Here is how that scenario would work if you were in touch with your frontal lobe. You're on the way to the gym when you see the side-walk sale, a trigger goes off to stop and check it out, and you activate the frontal lobe and look at the possibilities. It brings up an image in your head of the importance of working out. You weigh the consequences and benefits, and decide to follow through with your original plan of action. However, your frontal lobe starts to figure out a solution for you that will resolve the conflict. You decide that after you go to the gym, you will then go to the sidewalk sale and buy that outfit. In a nutshell, this is what happened. Your prefrontal cortex kept the images of the goal that you really wanted in your head. So your actions now matched your purpose of having that ideal, healthy body, and feeling great about yourself.

I have been practicing working with my frontal lobe so much that when I encounter such a scenario, the picture of what I really want stays in my mind. It becomes so real, so vivid that it feels like I am already there. This is when you really know that you're activating your frontal lobe. You often hear speakers talk about immediate gratification and long-term gratification. When the frontal lobe is at work, it will provide the inner strength to not respond to those stimuli that have us seeking immediate gratification. Instead of eating that ice cream cone or driving through the Mc-Donald's drive-thru, we have the ability to hold on to our long-term goals, dreams, aspirations, and purpose.

For most people who are overweight, one of the major causes of the extra pounds is a failure to work with the frontal lobe. An overweight person will easily be distracted, respond to an external stimulus, and overeat. We keep choosing the foods that are not good for us because we can recall what immediate pleasure they give us. We get so used to these familiar feelings that we crave more. The same response is triggered when we see an advertisement on TV for our favorite junk food, and we run out and get it. External stimuli in the environment trigger those familiar feelings in the body.

I am guilty of this as well. My weakness is theater popcorn—as large as you can get. If I know I am going to a movie that night, and if I am not careful, I could be creating pictures in my head all day of the popcorn that's producing the trigger in me. Even when I drive by a theatre, I notice my body completely changes. I notice I will say things like, "Could I ever go for some of that popcorn right now!" Simply the act of my seeing the movie theater sets off an external trigger that makes me want popcorn. If my frontal lobe does not go into action, I guarantee that every time I drive by a theatre, I will say, "Let's go to a movie," just so I can have popcorn.

Extreme concentrated focus

Through the frontal lobe you have extreme, concentrated focus; it's simply a matter of time before goals are achieved. The frontal lobe stops your brain from wandering off to other areas that prevent you from achieving your goals. When we see something in our environment that triggers an emotional reaction, the frontal lobe keeps us focused so we don't react to those emotions. As a result, you enjoy complete control over yourself.

Just as the Buddhist monks can quiet everything down, and are able to meditate at such a deep level, so too can we. When we're paying attention or focusing, we tend to get very still. We stop seeing the external world. Now something really amazing happens: because we have put the visual information coming in on pause, we now experience thoughts at a deeper level than we could ever imagine. Your thoughts take front and center stage in your mind. This also applies to your auditory cortex. You will no longer be aware of noises in the other room, other sounds. Everything starts to become quiet. Each and every one of these neurological signals is shut off by the frontal lobe. The noise that is running wild in your brain is turned right down. When all this works together, whatever we are focusing on or thinking about will become more real to us than the external world. The frontal lobe is so powerful that it can make a conscious thought so real that it seems as if nothing else exists.

The bottom line is a lot of us are overweight because of other events that are happening in our lives. If we are able to summon the power of the frontal lobe, we are able to tune out certain events that are not good for us. For example, say a family member yelled at you and you couldn't help thinking about it all day. Through the frontal lobe, we're able to tune out those events and get done what we need to get done in a day, such as going for a workout.

Let's face the facts: change is hard. Why? Because we seek comfort, and change means discomfort. Our old, boring, regular routine has hardwired our brain to the exact same neural networks that allow us to live that easy, comfortable, and always the same life. There go our dreams, our goals, and our inspirations to have that great, healthy body. Until you break out of the comfort zone, you're going to stay exactly where you are right now.

How many of us have repeated the exact same pattern for years? "I am going to start a new diet, an exercise program." "I am going to read a book a month." "I am not going to watch so much TV." "I am going to get up early and go to the gym." "I am going to prepare for my week in advance." You make all these plans only to find that all your aspirations get trampled by the circumstances that arise in life. All right, I think you now know enough about the frontal lobe, how it works, and just how important a part of your life these higher brain functions are.

Learn to observe yourself

What is the best way to put the frontal lobe to work for us? The first thing we have to do is observe ourselves. How do we know we have a problem if we can't see it? We don't. This is why many of us stay stuck in our old ways. I ask a lot of my clients to learn to observe themselves, their particular behaviors and personality traits. You can acquire this skill. It's the most important and easiest step to creating change.

If we can observe other people's behavior, then we can observe ourselves. We just have to open up our eyes and start looking. How many times have we looked at somebody else and thought, "I can't believe the way they're dressed," or, "I can't believe they chose that behavior. I would never do that!" "Can this person really see what he or she looks like?" The truth is, most likely not. They can see the larger world around them but they cannot clearly see themselves. They may spend a couple of hours in front of the TV every night, but they make no time in their life for self-reflection. They have no clue about the behavior they choose daily. They fail to ask themselves the right questions like, "Why do I keep producing these same negative emotions? Why is it that I expect one outcome but my behavior elicits a totally different response? Why is it that I keep getting the exact opposite of what I want in life? I want to be thin but I am fat. I want to be rich but I am poor. I want to have great feelings but I am down."

Once we activate the frontal lobe, we can start to see ourselves with great clarity. We stop responding to our external world and past memories. We eventually start to leave behind all the programs that we have been running that keep us emotionally addicted. I am not going to sugar-coat the process and say change is going to be easy. It's going to take some time, effort, and commitment. Your weight did not come on overnight. You did not become broke overnight. You did not establish bad emotions overnight. This all took some time to create. Conversely, it will take some time and commitment to change for the better.

So the first step is to become great observers of ourselves. In the same way that we observe other people, we need to step back and start observing ourselves to create lasting change.

Mental repetition

Now the next step is really going to start to employ the frontal lobe. This is where we need commitment. We need to set aside some time, and we need some dedication. If you follow this next step, which I call mental repetition, and you stick with it so it becomes a habit, you will start thinking like the heroes of the world. By using the mental repetition strategies that I set out for you, the frontal lobe will activate and you will start to make significant changes in your life.

The brain can't tell the difference between what's real and what's vividly imagined. So once we do something in our mind enough times, it becomes indistinguishable from doing it for real. Are you focused on exercising for life? Getting up early to achieve your goals? Becoming a more patient person? How about reducing stress? Success in mental repetition involves focusing on exactly what you want, and then visualizing yourself performing an action or skill in your mind. In terms of creating a change in ourselves, mental repetition is seeing ourselves in a certain situation, and becoming a different person or acting in a different way than how we previously would have acted.

Early in this chapter, I talked about how we get stuck in the thinking-and-feeling, feeling-and-thinking loop, which keeps us addicted to those emotional states and patterns we have run through over and over again. We need to be able to shift ourselves out of the thinking-and-feeling loop to get ourselves to take action and produce the results we're after in life. So here is the answer to breaking the cycle: activating the frontal lobe. When we have concentrated focus on a task at hand, it quiets the other parts of the brain, ending our pattern of thinking-and-feeling and feeling-and-thinking that keeps us addicted to certain emotional states.

You now can start to really think like the heroes of the world. The famous actor, Jim Carrey, one night drove his old Toyota up to Mulholland Drive in the Hollywood Hills, at the time a struggling Canadian comic trying to make it in the jungle of Los Angeles. As he sat high above the city, looking down, Carrey could see himself as one of the best actors of all time. Not only did he imagine himself being at the top, but he also wrote himself a check for $10 million, and added the notation, "for acting services rendered." He sat up on those hills not just once, but on many nights, visualizing himself as one of the best Hollywood actors ever. Yes, Jim Carrey was activating his frontal lobe, training his brain to produce maximum results. You can use the same strategies to produce results in your own life.

New knowledge

Learning new knowledge is a very important step. With new knowledge you can modify your old behavior and embrace new experiences. If we want to create change from the person we used to be, running the same patterns, we must not limit ourselves to beliefs we have stored in our brain, such as those that cause us to be overweight and out of shape. If you change your brain, you change your weight.

If you want new possibilities, you have to have new information. If you want to become a more motivated person, you have to do research on motivation. You may choose to think of a relative who was extremely motivated and note how they wrote down their goals, their positive attitude toward life, and the books they read. You can then take bits and pieces of what they did to achieve success, and use these lessons in your mental repetitions. There are countless ways you can learn new things, including through books, modeling successful people, informational TV or movies, exposure to new things, CDs, coaches, and seminars. The great thing is you're learning new knowledge right now just from reading this book.

The right environment

The next step to mental repetition is setting up the right environment. For maximum results, we need to get away from things that we're used to, the people, places, and things that make up our daily routines, that get us stuck in the exact same thought processes. I go to a little study room in my place that I rarely frequent otherwise. I light candles and play some soft music. Other times, I go to a secret place that overlooks my whole city of Vancouver. I go at night because I love to look at the lights that light up the whole sky for miles. Just like Jim Carrey, I look down on the city and do mental repetition on dreams and aspirations. It was not long ago that I sat up on that hill envisioning the lifestyle I wanted, the body I wanted, and the relationship I wanted. Today, those have all become my reality. I credit my success in achieving these goals to mental repetition.

Ask the right questions

Once you set up the environment that is going to best suit you, it's not enough to just sit down and visualize what you want. You also need to ask yourself certain intelligent questions, so your unconscious mind can come up with the answers. The right questions combined with mental repetition will fully activate the frontal lobe.

If we ask ourselves good quality questions, we get good results. If we ask ourselves poor quality questions, we get poor results. I see many people ask themselves poor questions that push them away from what they want; they start to attract what they don't want. Here are examples of some poor questions to ask yourself: "Is it too hot or too cold to exercise?" "Can I skip my workout today?" "Do I deserve a day off?" Here are some strong questions: "Won't it feel wonderful to achieve my fitness goals?" "How can I make this workout more fun?" "What music should I choose today during my workout?" "What foods will give me the most energy?" Can you see the difference in those questions?

Let me now give you some strong self-reflective questions you can ask yourself to help get the frontal lobe working to its fullest. Remember, you want to ask yourself good quality questions while doing your mental repetition. You can use these questions for all areas of your life.

- *What specifically do I want?*
- *How can I become better? (in a specific area)*
- *How can I modify my behavior? (regarding my weight, for example)*
- *How can I reinvent myself?*
- *What will this outcome allow me to do?*
- *How can I be different from how I am now?*
- *What do I have to change about myself to achieve a particular outcome?*
- *What is the highest vision of myself I can imagine?*
- *What's going to happen that gets me so excited?*
- *For what purpose do I want this?*
- *What behavior do I need to change to achieve my goal?*

- *What is (name the person) doing to achieve her goals and how can I replicate this success?*
- *How can I achieve more with less effort?*
- *What am I going to do to enjoy today?*
- *How good do I want to be at this?*
- *How can I get there in the quickest and most fun way?*

What I want you to do is write these questions down and eventually have them memorized. Every time you do mental repetition, you should be asking yourself these questions. Get into the habit for 30 days. Start to activate your frontal lobe, and I guarantee your weight and your life will completely change.

You don't have to ask all the questions in one sitting. Pick a few to focus on. Then, the next time you do mental repetition, pick different ones. If you're working to achieve your ideal, healthy weight, the questions should focus on your weight goal. You will be pleasantly surprised at how much this will help you change your life.

Make time for yourself

Have you ever said to yourself, "I just need some quiet time; I need some peace for a few moments?" It amazes me how many people say this and then make no time at all for themselves. One of my mentors runs 10 companies and various charities, and is always booked to speak, yet he still puts aside an hour a day to do mental repetition. So if you're saying you don't have the time, then I think you need to compare your schedule with his. Yes, he does have small kids as well, for those of you who are saying, "Well, I have kids." Don't make excuses; put aside the time to change your brain and your life.

The next step is to put aside 30 to 60 minutes per day to do mental repetition. Realize that if you mentally rehearse properly, that 30 to 60 minutes will seem like 5 minutes. All awareness of time and space will be absent. Your old state of being is probably trying to talk you out of change right now. "I don't have 30 minutes." "I'm so busy already." "My life is just the way I want it."

Don't fall into this trap again, the one you have been stuck in for years and years. Yes, you are now going to have to move out of your comfort zone. Think of the new patterns you're going to create just by setting aside 30 to 60 minutes per day for mental repetition. You will notice that from the repetition process alone your weight loss will speed up a great deal. You will start to become extremely focused and disciplined. You will reduce stress and become a very powerful person. You will start to feel that nothing can stop you from achieving your weight goal. In fact, you will start to feel that nothing can stop you from achieving any goal you set.

The best time to do mental repetition is first thing in the morning. If you can't seem to find the time first thing in the morning, make sure you find some time somewhere in the day. When we do this first thing in the morning, then when we walk out of the house, we start to act and think like that person we want to be. Our neural circuits in the brain are already warmed up. When we hit a challenge in our day, it's a lot easier to overcome that challenge since we're already thinking like the person we want to become.

So find a quiet spot and start focusing in on that person you want to become. Hold that vision of yourself in your mind. Eventually it will start to become more real than you ever possibly imagined. Do the repetitions for 30 days, focused on the new person you want to become or the new goals that you have in mind. Make sure you do mental repetitions for 30 days straight before you move onto something new. Let's say you want to be a more compassionate person or a healthy, in-shape person, focus on that one thing for 30 days straight. Then you can move on to some other behavior you would like to change or a goal you would like to achieve. It's also all right to repeat a goal or behavior for another 30 days, or to continue for longer than 30 days straight.

I am asking you to break the habits and patterns you have become emotionally addicted to, and start to practice what the new and improved you will be like. Whatever your vision is of that ideal self or the world you want to create, your commitment will ultimately pay off in ways that you have only begun to imagine. Now instead of just surviving, you can put yourself into a state of creation, just by activating your frontal lobe and changing your thinking. You can truly think and be like your heroes.

Do your mental repetition every day for at least 30-60 minutes, preferably in the morning, for 30 days straight. Then do another 30 days, and a third cycle of 30 days.

Congratulations!

NOTES:

CHAPTER SIX
The Connection Between Love and Weight Loss

Self-esteem, the subject we're going to cover in this chapter is, I believe, one of the most important on the planet. As important as it is, I find that people often overlook it, or do not take the time to figure out how it may be holding them back from a life of happiness, love, great health, and so much more.

The people I know who have mastered this subject really get to live a life that is out of this world. By the same token, the people who go through life and never truly master this concept are never truly fulfilled. They end up living a life of misery, with emotions up, down, and all around. Does this sound at all familiar?

The bottom line is this: having a healthy self-esteem, and having extremely high appreciation for yourself and even others, will give you the energy to truly fulfill your dreams. Having high self-esteem will take your weight and your health to a whole new level.

Too often when we get a little overweight, our weight goes up and our self-esteem goes down, and the appreciation we have for ourselves reaches an all-time low. It's not unlike your emotions. One minute you're happy and the next minute you're not quite sure why you're sad. It's the same with your self-esteem. One minute you're on top of the world, you have personal power and inner strength, you love yourself more than anybody else could ever love you, and then the next thing you know, your self-esteem is at an all-time low. You don't feel good about yourself, you're beating yourself up, you may even hate yourself, you start to dislike people around you, you feel you can't succeed, you start to get frustrated, and all the momentum you once had going is now completely gone.

Momentum is critical to success. But when you have low self-esteem or do not appreciate yourself, or even if you swing from high to low self-esteem, it is impossible to function optimally. Let me say it again: it is impossible to keep your momentum up, and it's impossible for you to succeed at your weight and health goals if you do not have high self-esteem.

Now you may be sitting there right now thinking to yourself, "I have the highest self-esteem. I don't need any help from you. I am just going to skip this chapter." Before you do that, I want you to stop and think again. You will learn techniques and strategies in this chapter that, even if you already have high self-esteem, will help take you to an even more profound level. Remember, there is not a person in this world who does not lose some of their self-esteem at times.

So what is this thing we call self-esteem? Basically, it's how you see yourself, and how that view influences all of your experiences. It's the basic requirement for peace of mind and personal satisfaction.

Can you remember a time in your life when you were "on fire" and felt great about yourself? Go back right now and experience that time. See what you were seeing, feel what you were feeling. Maybe there were sounds you were hearing. Now stop and notice how you feel right now. How good do you feel?

Now what would happen if you had the power to choose that state at any time in your life? What if you could go back and instantly – as fast as you can snap your fingers – start to experience those exact same feelings again? What if at any time you could go back and love yourself more than you could possibly imagine?

Now go back and remember a time when you did not feel good about yourself. You may have been beating yourself up, not loving yourself, talking negatively to yourself; maybe your self-esteem was at an all-time low. Go back and really remember what you were seeing, the sounds you were hearing, the feelings you were experiencing. What were you feeling when your self-esteem and self appreciation were at an all-time low?

So what stops you from choosing a healthy self-esteem? The problem is most people don't choose high or low self-esteem, it chooses you. The next question then would be, why does it choose you? Is low self-esteem just a monster that decides to choose you? Not likely. It chooses whom it chooses simply because most people have no idea how to create high self-esteem.

I am going to teach you some in-depth but easy to follow techniques that can help you change certain behaviors when it comes to self-esteem. These techniques will help skyrocket your success and take your self-appreciation to the next level. Many people think that to change your self-esteem, you need a massive amount of willpower, that that's the only way it's ever going to work. That's completely wrong. Any time you're going to create any changes in your life, willpower alone will never work.

Think about this: How much willpower did you use to create low self-esteem? You probably sat there all night trying your hardest to create low self-esteem. You probably kept saying to yourself for days and days, "I do not love myself. I am not a great person. I can never succeed." For two days you did this, and for some reason, it just did not work. Five more days went by, and you tried so hard to create low self-esteem.

So did it happen? No, of course not. You did not have to use a massive amount of willpower to create low self-esteem. It just seemed to happen. It was actually quite easy for you to create it. You did not have to use willpower at all. You were already trained and most likely quite proficient at this skill, a skill that we have to make it a priority to change.

You can have all the willpower in the world and still not create a great picture of yourself, a view that positively influences all of your experiences. Using willpower will actually create frustration and bring on more and more low self-esteem because it just does not work. Your self-esteem is not a reflection of who you actually are, but an internal representation of yourself, and the way you think and talk to and about yourself.

Change these two things – your internal representations and your self-talk – and you can literally change your self-esteem. A person's self-image is defined by the intensity of the visual submodalities (the specific characteristics of the visual image) that you're running in your brain. Let's take an image that's dark, small, and far away. Now let's take an image that's bright and near. Which image is going to be more attractive? Of course, the one that's bright and near. Low self-esteem is very often linked to a very intense, negative self-image.

For example, Kathy, a weight loss client of mine, found herself unable to attain her ideal, healthy weight when she knew she was fully capable. She had done it before, but this time she seemed not to be able to stay on track. When we sat down and took a look at her internal representations, Kathy discovered that she was producing a self-image that was negative and upsetting. She was overweight, feeling unattractive, and never able to succeed. She literally saw this vividly colored snapshot – big, bright, and extremely close to her face. The content of her self-image was very disturbing to look at, and the intensity was at an all-time high, too close in her mind.

Every time Kathy thought of her self-worth she would start to feel less and less positive in regard to herself. Even when she was losing weight, she was still portraying that same negative outlook and engaging in negative self-talk. She could not see herself as a healthy, in-shape person. Other people would even tell her, "You look like you've lost weight and you look great!" But the images she was seeing were still of herself as overweight, ugly, and unhealthy. Each time she put herself into a disempowering emotional state, she could tell she was starting to go back to the mindset of thinking like an overweight person. The combination of the negative content and its intensity left Kathy feeling helpless.

To be able to create change, we had to go back and look at what was going on in Kathy's brain when she was in great shape, happy, and healthy. When Kathy was at her best, she would see herself as a very confident, happy, energetic person. The images in her mind were that of a positive Kathy that would motivate her and help her attain her goals. We did some manipulation with her visual sub-modalities, and the next thing you know, she was back to being a confident, happy, motivated person. She has now lost over forty-five pounds.

There are different levels of self-esteem: high, low, medium, and medium negative self-esteem. High self-esteem has very positive content in an intense form. Low self-esteem has very negative content in an intense form. Medium self-esteem is seeing your self-image in a medium intensity form. You can change this just by changing the submodalities (the qualities of the images in your head), making them brighter, more colorful, closer, in motion, or whatever would make that image more attractive for you. The positive content would stay exactly the same, but the form would be made that much more attractive. Medium negative self-esteem appears in the form of a medium negative self-image. To change it, and shift into having high self-esteem, both content and form need to be changed.

The pictures that we run in our brain can be extremely negative or extremely positive. Anybody who is overweight and gets into great shape has learned how to change the pictures and, therefore, their self-image.

When it comes to your weight, it does not matter how overweight you are right now. You may be thinking, "What are you talking about Shane?" But it does not matter, be-cause today is a brand new day. That means you can be a brand new you; it does not matter what has happened in the past. Who you decide to become today is what is going to shape your character and, therefore, shape your future.

Many times when it comes to our self-esteem, we look outside ourselves. What I mean by that is, we see ourselves as an outside observer, imagining how someone else might see us. Then that view becomes our belief of who we are. But a much more effective technique is to start seeing yourself through the eyes of someone who loves you. People often see us differently from how we see ourselves, and loved ones often see things that we don't.

Powerful Self-Esteem Exercise

This exercise can really be enlightening by helping you to see yourself the way a loved one would see you.

First, find a comfortable and quiet place. All right, start to relax. Breathe in and out slowly. Take another big breath in, and now let it out. Very good. Another breath in, and now let it all out. Very good.

- What I want you to do is think of someone who loves you. Think of someone who without a doubt loves you. It could be your partner, friend, lover, child, grandparent, aunt, or uncle. If you are unable to think of a person who loves you, then think of a person who has assisted you along the way, and you know that this person really appreciates you. Either it's someone you know loves you or someone you know deeply appreciates you. In either case, simply notice who he or she is for now.

- Now you're going to design an autobiography. What I want you to do is imagine you're writing your autobiography. You're very relaxed and comfortable as you're writing your autobiography. You can imagine exactly where you're sitting as you write.

- You may realize, right away, in a few seconds or maybe later on, how the words that describe your life begin to easily occur to you. And as you write, you become alert of the thoughts of person who loves you... or respects you. You start to think even more clearly about that individual who you know loves you.

- Now see the person you know loves you. Take your time to see him or her. Look across the room from where you're writing your autobiography, you can see the person on the other side of the glass door, the person that you know loves you. As you focus on this someone who you know loves you or appreciates you, you become aware that he or she is starring at you, observing you. And you decide to write about this person and the role he or she has played in your life in your autobiography. Take a minute and describe this someone, what you vision and what you feel about this someone. Even describe what you hear yourself saying about this person who you know loves you. Write all this in your autobiography.

- See yourself from another perspective. Now that you have a full sense of what it's like to describe the person who you know loves you, allow yourself to float outside your body at the desk and float your awareness through the room out the glass door, and recognize what it's like to stand next to the someone who cares you as you are writing. Just notice what you look like from this awareness of being behind the glass door. And notice how much you currently love yourself. Recognize your actual feelings about yourself as you see yourself through the glass door. You may recognize a vast amount of self-appreciation, or you may only see a little. Whatever you recognize, simply accept this experience.

- Recognize yourself through the eyes of someone who loves you deeply. Now, enter into the body of the person who you know loves you deeply. Do this in a relaxing and slow way. And when you are fully in the body of the person who you know loves and appreciates you, see through the person's eyes at yourself as you design your autobiography. Picture yourself through the eyes of someone who appreciates you. See what you look like writing your autobiography. And notice the actions you take.

- Fully accept the qualities and special attributes of yourself that you are aware of, perhaps this is the first time, as you recognize yourself through the eyes of love. And because you're in the body of a person who loves you, become aware of the thoughts you capture being said about you and the feelings being felt about you. Recognize the tone of speech of the positive, uplifting thoughts you hear as you see yourself over there, writing at your peaceful desk, from the eyes of someone who you know loves you.

- Come back to your own perspective. When you are fully engaged of the qualities and important aspects of yourself that make you who and what you are, allow your perspective to leave the body of the someone who you know loves you deeply, and float back through the glass door gently, and back inside your body at the desk writing your autobiography.

- Write about your out of body experience. Please take your time and write into your autobiography experiencing yourself through the eyes of love or appreciation. As you write about you're out of body experience, please list several of the qualities and important aspects you recognized in yourself when you saw yourself through the eyes of love.

- Look into the future. As you write, look into your future, both of future experiences you understand

are coming, and become aware of those unexpected experiences that might surprise you. Think
of all the events and places, and days and even
years from now, when you'll safely be able to review, recall, and remember this amazing experience of seeing yourself through your eyes of love,
noticing your uniqueness and deeply loving who
and what you are in the world.

• Return to this moment. Now, become fully aware,
your full consciousness. At your own speed, become awake and alert. Now come back to this
present moment and place, feeling better than
ever. Hear the sounds in the room. And you can
recognize the feelings in your body. And in a second, you can open your eyes as you slowly return
to your full conscious awareness and stretch your
body.

• Notice the difference. Now you have had the
luxury to easily experience the self-appreciation
that eludes so many people. Recognize how this
exercise has changed the picture of yourself in
moderate and not so moderate ways. Recognize
how you can now actually picture yourself from a
new, happier, and loving perspective. The experience you have just received has provided you with
strong personal self-appreciation that is a fast
step toward supporting, loving and encouraging
yourself.

There is a very simple but profound way that you can
build your self-esteem every day at any time. Most people
I know that have extremely high self-esteem consistently
use this technique. Just one word can literally change your
self-esteem in seconds. The key is to use an I statement
or an I am statement.

For example, you could say "I am in great shape!" You
may be overweight, but the brain can't tell the difference.

This is helpful because you put yourself into positive emotional states, and when you're in these uplifting states, that's when you're motivated to work out, eat healthy and, even more importantly, become aware of your thinking patterns.

Most of us just turn off our brains. Why? Because thinking is the hardest job in the world. But that's exactly what this program is designed to do, get you thinking, noticing what's going on in your head instead of just going through life completely unaware. When you make the choice to start making I statements and I am statements, your weight will change, your self-esteem will change, your life will change.

So say to yourself right now, "I love myself." Come on, say it again. "I love myself." One more time. "I love myself." I know right now you might be having a hard time saying that. You're not used to telling yourself that you love yourself. You are probably better at telling other people you love them than actually telling yourself that you love yourself.

Let's try this again. Say to yourself, "I am awesome." Come on, yell it out. "I am awesome!" Now pump your fist when you yell, "I am awesome!" Did you pump your fist? Get that right into your nervous system. When you get your body involved as you say something, it's a lot easier to feel it. And remember, what you feel is what you will think.

I statements are great for giving you ownership of all your actions. When you use an I statement, you're standing up for yourself and your identity. You brain will start to say, "I am a great person. I am myself, I am this person that loves myself, and am no one else. I know I may have imperfections, little quirks, but I love myself because I am a great person. I am special, I am unique, I am wonderful." Nobody can take this away from you.

Just the act of being born on this planet makes you special and unique. You are a gift, and I am grateful to be able to work with you. I love you and care about you deeply even though I don't know you personally. I feel like I do, and I just want to say congratulations for following through with this program.

If you watch good leaders, you will see they have extremely high self-esteem. So what allows these people to have such high self-esteem and lead the way they lead? Are they born with it? Do they have a gift from god? No, they have just developed the ability to solidify their own identity. They don't take other people's identity away from them, but allow others to have their own beliefs, opinions, and differences. They feel very safe with themselves and others, and they're not afraid to separate themselves with their own visions, ideas, dreams, goals, feelings, and values. They allow themselves to express themselves, and to be different just by being who they are.

A good leader has the ability to say yes or no. If a leader did not have the ability to say no, every yes would be totally meaningless. If you consistently say yes, this takes away your freedom of choice, and will lower your self-esteem as a result of not being able to choose your own life. I see this happen all the time when people have low self-esteem.

Let's take an example that many of you will be able to relate to. You have been working for two months to get your mind right. You're on track; you're really making it happen. You're working out, eating healthy, you're in a good emotional state and are on fire for success in your life. We have all had a time in our life when everything just seemed to flow.

Christmas comes along, and you say to yourself, "I am not going to go out and overeat. I am going to say no to those crappy foods. I have set my mind right. I am going to do it this time." You're feeling motivated and strong.

Everyone shows up for Christmas, the goodies come out, and you say no. You hear your sister asking if you're on a diet. She's telling you it's Christmas and it's okay for you to have a little bite! You stay strong, and you say no. From the back of the room you hear someone make a small comment about your eating. You choose to ignore it. Dinner comes along. You do well, you don't overeat, you choose healthy foods, and you feel great about yourself. Now dessert comes along: the pie, the goodies; everyone starts passing them around. You decline, but everyone is asking why, and if you're on a diet, or perhaps saying it's okay to cheat on Christmas.

Finally, you just cave. You can't handle it anymore. Your brain says you want the pie. At that moment it tastes so good, but as soon as you're done, you start to become aware of your thinking process.

This has everything to do with your self-esteem. Whenever you're pressured by other people and you cave in to what you don't really want to do, it is a sign of low self-esteem. Now you can change this. How do you change a habit? You do the exact opposite. You have to become consciously aware of when this is happening, and learn to say no in these situations. As you become accustomed to saying no, you will notice your self-esteem getting stronger and stronger. Eventually, you will be so strong and powerful that you will be able to say no at any time when someone tries to force you to do something you do not want to do.

This works both ways: if you're not able to say no, and say yes all the time, or if you're not able to say yes, and say no all the time. Just remember not to sacrifice your beliefs, dreams, goals, and especially your values for anyone else. Low self-esteem plays a big role in your weight because overeating is an addiction. If you have high self-esteem, you're not going to harm your body. The same is true with addictive, compulsive behaviors and co-dependency.

I find that one of the most detrimental influences on the self-esteem of overweight people is their fear of criticism.

If they are criticized, they have no idea how to handle it. But this is not just a major issue for overweight people; it's a big issue for many people across the world in all areas of life. Criticism can break down your self-esteem faster than you can take a breath in, but once you learn how to deal with it, you can build your self-esteem faster than you can absorb the criticism.

The first thing I think is important for you to realize about criticism is that every behavior is useful in some context. Now you may be sitting there thinking that I have totally lost my marbles. How could this be? Bear with me, and let me explain.

The fear of criticism and of rejection can hold us back from having the body and the life we have always wanted. I had a lady in one of my weight loss seminars stand up and say: I just realized why I am so scared of rejection. When I was a teenager, I was extremely overweight, and so were my two sisters. When I turned 17, I lost all of my excess weight, and was starting to look and feel really good. From that time, my sisters started rejecting me. They wanted nothing to do with me. I gained the weight back so I would no longer be rejected by them. To this day, I will do anything to avoid those feelings of rejection. That's what's been holding me back for so long in my life. I don't even really want to get rid of my excess weight because I am so scared I will be rejected again. So I eat and eat, and would rather be fat than have that feeling of rejection.

She said she had to share her story because for the last two days at the seminar she had started to eat healthy again, as she was no longer afraid of rejection. By the way, she has now lost 85 pounds, and has an incredible new man in her life.

Can you believe that we can make such strong associations with emotions connected to past events that it stops us from succeeding? Once you have taken action to control this emotion, rejection is something that you will never have to fear again. Whatever you set your mind to you will achieve. Make yourself feel powerful. Make it very hard to feel rejection. Everyone has a right to their way of thinking, but if you don't agree with them, you don't have to feel badly. It's important to touch on the fear of rejection in more depth because if you can overcome that fear in every area of your life, your self-esteem will be at an all-time high.

Fear of Rejection

Fear stops us from doing many things. Fear operates as a powerful force in everyone's life. Of all the emotions, the one emotion that people will do just about anything to avoid is this little word we call rejection. The word rejection just scares the wits right out of people. What makes you feel rejected? There is nothing — no event or experience or person outside of you — that can make you feel rejected. You're the only one that can generate this painful emotion inside of you. Rejection is just something you create in your brain. You give yourself the triggers that set it off.

I want you to get control over yourself. So ask yourself the following questions: What is the price that you will pay if you do not take control of this emotion called rejection? What opportunities are you going to miss out on? How many people are you not going to meet? What will your health be like? What will your self-esteem be like? How much money are you going to let pass you by? What kind of friendships are you going to miss out on? If you don't handle this fear of rejection, what is the price you're going to pay for long-term results in your life?

Make a list of all the benefits that would happen in your life if you could free yourself from this fear of rejection. Imagine if you could not feel anxiety, not have the chattering of the monkey in your mind holding you back, but instead be 100 percent free and clear of it. Imagine that whatever you want you constantly keep going after until you get it. What kind of confidence do you think you would gain? What courage would you develop? What kind of success could you have? What action would you be consistently taking? What you must do is really get yourself to buy into the extraordinary results you're going to get from overcoming this fear of rejection.

Outline enough reasons so that when you are dealing with feelings of rejection, your brain links up to the negative and positive outcomes. The end goal is to see the benefits of overcoming the feelings of rejection, and get ready to create that change. You need enough reasons to encourage your brain to say: This is going to take me to the next level of my life. I know all the wonderful things that can happen in my life. This is what I have to do to succeed.

What you want to do now is create a new set of principles that have to happen for you to feel rejected. For example, right now the principles for you to feel rejected may be, you call up a billionaire and he says, "No, I will not mentor you." It's like he's not giving you his approval, and you feel rejected. Or you tell someone your goal of how much weight you're going to lose and they say, "Yeah right, you're never going to do it." Again, you feel like you're not getting the approval you seek and you feel rejected. Many times when it comes to our weight, we're looking for approval from other people. You are setting yourself up to be rejected.

So what we have to do is to change your principles. Just think if you had principles established to help you succeed even when someone tried to make you feel rejected. Maybe the only time you would feel the emotion of rejection is when you knew somebody was right. It's extremely important to come up with a great principle for yourself, so no one can make you feel rejected.

The first thing you have to realize is that you must make the decision to not let anyone's opinion destroy the way you feel about yourself. Now think about this: if you refuse to accept someone's abuse, you choose not to play the game. The abuse they are giving you still belongs to them. There will be times in your life, actually a lot of times, when you will be dealing with people who may be in a bad state that day. They may be in a state of stress, or anger, or frustration. You ask for something and they reject you. It's just because of the state they're in at that time. They may not be rejecting you; they're just in a rejecting state. So don't ever allow this to affect you.

Create a new set of principles for yourself. Make it hard to feel rejected, raise your level for success, step up into the next level, and see what happens. How do you create a new set of principles for yourself? Make sure your principles support you on the road to personal growth and do not limit you. Realize that people are not rejecting you. They may be rejecting your idea or they're rejecting how they see you in this moment; they're not rejecting everything about you, who you are, what you stand for. They're rejecting one specific thing, and the whole you is much more than that.

Can you remember a time when you did not initially like somebody, but then you grew to like them, and you actually started becoming really good friends? See, when you meet someone for the first time and they don't respond to you the way you want, or they express feelings as if they don't like you, it is not a permanent thing. It could be just the state they are in at that time. It's just their behavior in that moment. As time goes on, they could very well end up liking you a lot. Unless you take it personally and communicate at a low level and, as a result, fail to get through to others.

All right, so you set up some new principles for yourself. What are some other ways to handle rejection? Massively failing is another key to success. Okay, okay, before you think I have totally lost my mind, let me explain.

This is the hardest principle for most people to get, but if you can truly get this, I mean, if you can link this into your nervous system, you will massively succeed by massively failing. Think about this: If you're not being rejected, you're not becoming successful. The world's most successful people have been rejected far more than they have succeeded. Anyone who has succeeded has gone through massive rejection. Continually taking action toward what you want will eliminate your fear of rejection.

Another approach that I have used myself for years is that I have conditioned myself to enjoy rejection. So just how do you do that? Well, the exact same way you condition yourself to feel crappy. You have to create a new neural connection. What I have done for myself and others is created an anchor so strong that when someone rejects me, I automatically go into a state of joy and success. I feel the feelings of getting closer to my goals.

Exercise:

Put yourself into a state where you feel incredibly strong, where you feel unstoppable, like you can accomplish anything you set your mind to. The truth is you can accomplish anything you set your mind to once you decide to do it. So once you get into the state of feeling strong, do it over and over again. Remember, you have to stand and breathe in alignment with that powerful state, and you have to be fully associated for this to work. Picture yourself having a strong, healthy body, looking good, feeling good, and having all the confidence in the world.

Rehearse in your mind someone rejecting you and, in response, you feel stronger and stronger. The more the person rejects you, the stronger you get. Pick a role model. It may be Donald Trump, Richard Branson, Martha Stewart, a famous sports star, elite motivational speaker, or Oprah. Imagine that your role model has taken over your body, and no matter what this person does to reject you, you still get them to mentor you. Watch what Oprah, or Donald, or whomever you picked, does with their body, their face, and their voice to make all this happen. The more rejection you get, the more committed you are to securing a mentorship with some of the world's most successful people.

Allow rejection to drive you. Enjoy rejection because you know that you're getting closer to what you want. You're stepping up to the next level. No rejection equals no success. You can choose to overcome any form of rejection. How you perceive yourself is how most people are going to respond to you. If your own perception of yourself on the inside is powerful, it will radiate outside of you, and you will attract everything you need.

Write down three instances where you have been rejected in your life.

Write down what benefits you received from being rejected.

I want you remember a time when you were rejected, one of those times that has really stuck with you. It may have affected you at a deep level. It could go back as far as your childhood.

Now I want you to stand up, and stand as if you were the richest and healthiest person in the world. Hold yourself as if you have tremendous energy and excitement that spreads around the whole room. I want you to breathe the way you would breathe when you feel like you're on fire, like you can succeed at anything, like you're powerful, unstoppable, and proud. Breathe this way and feel this way. Now that you're feeling really powerful, I want you to create a positive anchor. So when you're at your peak of feeling powerful, do something unique. Do something unique over and over again, so that when you do this later on, you can feel this positive feeling again. Pump your fist in the air, or just do something so you feel really good. Do it again and link it to something. Feel good and link it to something.

Okay, now that you're feeling powerful, let's do the following:

Remember that time when you got rejected? Imagine that you're watching it on a movie screen in front of you. I want you to watch the movie one time exactly the way it happened. I want you to make sure you stay in that powerful state as you watch it go across the screen. Watch how you experienced it back then. You may feel some of the feelings you felt back then, but they won't be as intense because they're outside of you. Keep watching it, all the way, until you start to come to the end of the movie, the place where you felt bad because you were rejected.

Now, standing tall, again feeling really powerful, I want you to get a little crazy, a little playful, like you're a little kid again. Get excited. Go for it! Be a little crazy, and have a little fun. Now what I want you to do is put a smile on your face, close your eyes, and remember that same memory, but this time start at the end of that memory. When I say go, I want you to run that entire memory backwards in time, as fast as you possibly can. See everything you did moving in reverse. As you are talking, the words are coming right back into your mouth. While you're doing this, I want you to see your favorite colors around everywhere. You may even hear some weird noises going on.

Ready, go! All the way to the beginning, as fast as you possibly can. And if there are people rejecting you, watch them develop Mickey Mouse ears, and see their noses grow like Pinocchio.

Now run the movie forward again, but run it twice as fast. If there is anybody around you that's rejecting you, watch them shrink down and kneel down. Whisper to them, "It's okay." See the same memory as fast as you can, faster, faster, faster. Make it all kinds of different colors. Their ears are growing like Mickey Mouse. Their nose is getting long like Pinocchio. Watch them shrink down, and kneel down and tell them, "It's okay." See the sun shining on their faces. Imagine all kinds of crazy pictures flashing by you all the way to the end.

Okay, stop. You should be right back at the end. Now you're going to run it backwards as fast as you can go, but listen to your favorite music. Watch the movie in reverse, everything moving in reverse, fast, fast, fast. Now go forward again. Do this four times back and forth, back and forth – fast, fast, fast. Each time change something so it's a little bit different. Make it a little more crazy. Make the whole thing black and white. Now place the whole thing in a big ray of sunshine.

All right. Put a smile on your face, and go back and remember that memory of rejection. What happens now? Maybe you see a Pinocchio or sunshine. Do you feel aligned? If not, run this pattern over and over. All we're doing is interrupting the pattern.

What happens if you get rejected again? First, see what you can learn from it. Then use this technique to get rid of the negative feelings. Don't play the same memory over and over, and keep saying the same things to yourself over and over. If you keep picturing the same things, you're going to keep getting the same results.

If you use this technique, it will completely change your life. The key to successful weight loss and a successful life is to make sure you take action on everything I teach, and apply the strategies day in and day out. You will get massive rewards.

Action Steps

Describe what having a healthy self-esteem will do for you as a person:

_____

_____

_____

_____

What steps can you take today to build your self- esteem?

_____

_____

_____

_____

NOTES:

CHAPTER SEVEN
Eating To Increase Your Life Span And Reduce Your Waistband

What is your philosophy on health? What beliefs have you taken on about what causes disease in the body and what creates optimal health? What is your foundation for creating great health? The perspective that you take towards your health can be the most important decision you ever make in your life. Do you really know where your beliefs come from regarding vital health? Most of us have taken very little time to examine the choices we make when it comes to our overall health.

The biggest obstacle I see when it comes to a life of vitality and health is that most of our beliefs are formed unconsciously. We hear some piece of information from an advertiser, a friend, a family member, government bodies, or medical professionals, and we implant that information into our data bank and hold it as true, without evaluating it first. This would be alright if everybody acted with good intentions in this world, if they did and said things that had your best interests in mind. However, this is not always the case. You must first make an intelligent, educated decision before adopting some of these beliefs and ideas. Take the weight loss industry as one example. Every time a new program comes along, it is often designed to give you a quick fix. Do you think these companies have your best interests in mind for your overall health? Do you think when a drug company produces a commercial that there is no financial gain for them? I am not saying information is bad, but the information you take in should be evaluated with common sense, and it should have a proven track record. We must take control of the decisions we make about our health.

Question everything; leave nothing to chance

In the area of health, what beliefs do you hold as true right now? How do these beliefs serve you? What if you were able to open your mind, let go of your convictions, and expand yourself with new information so you can make new choices?

What is great health?

Science says that great health means a person has energy, feels well, and is free of illness. I would define health as a state of well-being – mentally, physically, emotionally and socially. It's not just the absence of disease in the body, but having an abundance of healthy energy.

Healthy cells create a healthy body

The energy your body needs is derived from the metabolic processes that take place in your cells. Cells are the building blocks of your life, and the quality of your health is dependent on the quality of your cells. It is estimated that the body can have as many as 100 trillion cells. Each one of these cells has a specific job to carry out. Take, for example, your red blood cells. The job of the red blood cells is to carry oxygen to cells throughout the body. Each cell's job is essential for keeping the body alive and healthy. Without healthy cells, you will have a poor quality of life.

As the image on the next page shows, bone cells differ from blood cells, and nerve cells differ from muscle cells. Each cell is designed to do a different job. Nerve cells carry electrical signals to and from the brains and muscles throughout the body. Red blood cells carry oxygen. Bone cells, which are very rigid, form the skeleton that gives the body shape. Muscle cells contract to move the bones and give us mobility. Stomach cells secrete an acid to digest

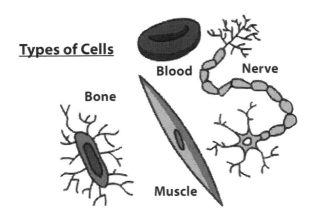

Types of Cells

Blood

Nerve

Bone

Muscle

our food. Cells in our intestines absorb nutrients from the food we eat. The one thing these cells all have in common is that they change nutrients into energy to keep us alive.

How to have healthy cells

Healthy mental attitude

Positive, peaceful thoughts, emotions, beliefs, and attitudes have a huge effect on our cells. When you remove the stress from your life, and provide the body with energy, the cells and body start to heal themselves. The natural state of the body's cells is peace, balance, harmony, and ease. This is a good way to understand the word health: the body's natural state when the cells are not stressed.

Exercise, deep breathing, and your cells

Exercise and deep breathing are critical to maintaining healthy cells and a healthy body. When you exercise, you help oxygenate the cells and, in return, your cells start to work at an optimum level. And research has shown that the best way to get the lymphatic system working is through deep breathing.

Let me explain the lymphatic system more in-depth. Lymph vessels form a drainage system throughout the body. The lymphatic fluid carries away the debris of our immune system, including dead white blood cells, unused plasma protein, and toxins. The heart pumps blood around the body, transporting nutrients and oxygen to the cells. The cells then absorb what they need, and excrete debris and toxins, which are then flushed out and deactivated by the lymphatic fluid. This lymphatic fluid drains into the circulatory system and becomes part of the blood and plasma that pass through the kidneys and liver.

The lymphatic system does not have a built-in pump like the heart. It relies on breathing and movement to circulate all that fluid and remove waste. When you have a poorly functioning lymphatic system, your body cannot detoxify properly. If your lymphatic fluid is not flowing as well as it should, then you are not breathing properly and moving your body enough.

The consequences are weight gain, muscle loss, high blood pressure, loss of energy, and inflammation. Just by expanding and contracting your diaphragm, you can stimulate the lymphatic system and send signals to the internal organs, helping the body to rid itself of toxins and leave more room in the cells for optimal levels of oxygen. It is extremely important to exercise and do breathing exercises to keep your cells healthy.

Cell protection

One of the most important things a cell needs to protect itself from all the toxins flowing through the body is to have the ability to eliminate waste efficiently. Blood carries body wastes from the cells to the kidneys and the lungs, the organs that eliminate wastes from the body. In the kidneys, cell wastes are filtered out of the body and excreted in the urine. In the lungs, carbon dioxide, a product of respiration, is removed from the blood and expelled when you breathe out.

The best way to fight disease in the body is to have a strong, healthy immune system. Those who maintain their immune system at optimal performance are more likely to avoid pharmaceutical drugs, surgery, and all the other complications that come with having a weak immune system. Science has shown that we are only as healthy as our cells. We only grow old when our cells grow old.

Environmental pollutants and your cells

Our cells need to have as much clean air and clean water as we can get for them to work well. The air we breathe is polluted with toxic emissions from vehicles, chemicals from factories, heavy metals from cigarettes, smoke, dust, and chemicals from appliances such as air conditioners and refrigerators. The fact is, there are pollutants in our environment you cannot avoid, unless you want to move to a secluded island, which may just be your best choice. For most of us, however, this is not a realistic option.

The water we bathe in and drink is usually no better than the air we breathe. It contains chlorine, heavy metals, toxic, organic chemicals from factories, pesticides, and herbicides. The water we drink plays an important role in the detoxification of our cells and in cellular nutrition. Cells have to be well hydrated for the proper elimination of toxins and assimilation of nutrients.

What creates a healthy environment for the cells in the body? Proper water intake — good, clean water, not tap water or impure bottled water — is one of the most important aspects of good health. It raises your pH balance so that your body stays alkaline. A cell will become unhealthy when there's an imbalance in the cell's environment. An acidic environment can lead to the development of diseases, including cancer.

Chlorophyll

One of the best cellular detoxifying agents is chlorella. Only chlorella contains a "high-fiber cell wall", that researchers have shown to be capable of removing heavy metals, such as mercury, cadmium, nickel, and lead, from the body. It is also capable of removing toxic chemicals such as dioxins and PCBs. Chlorella performs a function no other whole food can.

Significantly, chlorella is very rich in chlorophyll, a natural cleanser that is acknowledged as the best detoxifying agent for the cells of the body. It has been shown to remove chemicals such as pesticides, herbicides, and other toxic organic chemicals. Chlorophyll also cleanses the blood, helping to keep cells clean. Besides its potent detoxifying properties, chlorella is also rich in Chlorella Growth Factor (CGF), which helps revitalize and rejuvenate the cells. CGF is high in RNA and DNA, and is touted as an anti-aging factor.

Oxygen is vital for energy

What is the most critical element that our cells require in order to operate at their best? To live a life full of energy and vitality, you need adequate oxygen. The problem is most of us do not get sufficient amounts of oxygen. According to NASA, which ensures that astronauts have enough oxygen in space, the average person requires 0.84 kg of oxygen per day. Most of us are taking in less than half of our required daily intake of oxygen. If you take in more oxygen, you will notice a definite change in the quality of your life.

Oxygen generates a molecule in the body called ATP.

The body needs ATP to survive; it is the engine that powers all of the cell's activities. Think about what you are doing when you breathe. You are taking in oxygen, and that oxygen generates energy.

When you take in too much food, your body has trouble digesting all of it, so your energy level decreases. As a result, your body has trouble eliminating the toxins swimming around in your system. Your body then holds onto more water and fat. When you have excess water and fat in your system, there is less space in between your cells. And if you have less space in between your cells, you have less oxygen. If we stay on this same track, our body eventually starts to break down, our looks start to fade, our energy levels deplete, and maintaining our overall health becomes a constant struggle.

To prevent this from happening, we have to get our lymphatic system working. Think about your lymphatic system like your heart; your heart is the pump that keeps everything moving. To stay alive and healthy, you need to pump your lymphatic system by moving. If you don't move, the lymph system cannot cleanse your body. You actually have more lymphatic fluid in your body than you do blood. The key is to keep that lymphatic fluid moving, and you are the pump.

It is critical that you move. But even more importantly, research has shown that the best way to get the lymphatic system working optimally is through deep breathing. Most of us don't breathe properly throughout the day. Master correct breathing and you will keep your lymphatic system pumping.

Cleansing breath

1. Breathe normally, in through your nose and out through your mouth.

2. When you breathe, clear your lungs completely by pushing out the last part of the breath in short spurts through your mouth.

3. Take a deep breath through your nose, using your diaphragm to pull your lungs down and outward (rather than pushing your chest out and shoulders back).

4. Release your breath slowly.

5. Clear your lungs completely, and breathe using the 1-4-2 ratio. Breathe in for 1 count, hold for 4 counts, and exhale for 2 counts.

6. Now breathe in for 4 counts, hold for 16 counts, and release for 8 counts. Try it one more time.

As your lung capacity increases, you will be able to breathe in for a longer period of time. For example, breathe in for 8 counts, hold for 32 counts, and release for 16 counts. Repeat this routine 3 times per day. Do this when you awake in the morning, after you have had your glass of water, and twice more throughout the day. This will not take very long.

This is such an easy process to increase your energy, fight off toxins, and live a much longer, healthier life. Now that you realize the power of the breath, your job is to take action and follow through. I can only give you the knowledge. You have to do the doing part, and then you will shift into the being part. You will have taken on a new life habit. The being part is when you have mastered it, when it becomes part of your everyday lifestyle.

Quality water

What causes you to be dehydrated?

Without oxygen, we will die within minutes. Without food, an adult can live several weeks. And without water, we can survive about 10 days. Water is essential to human life. It forms the basis for all bodily fluids, including blood and digestive juices; it helps eliminate waste; and it assists in the transportation and absorption of all our nutrients. Water is the single largest component of the body: the brain is 76% water, blood is 84% water, the lungs are 90% water, and blood plasma is 98% water.

The average adult loses more than 10 cups (close to 2.5 liters) of water every single day, simply by sweating, breathing, and eliminating waste. We generally replace this lost water through the fluids we drink and the food we eat. But when you eliminate more water and salts than you replace, dehydration sets in – your system literally dries up. Even in a state of mild dehydration, things like fatigue, decreased coordination, and loss of judgment will set in. You will also lose minerals such as sodium, potassium, and calcium that maintain the balance of fluids in your body. Don't let yourself fall into the trap of not drinking enough water because you are sick, busy, or because you lack access to good quality water while traveling.

Warning signs of dehydration

The U.S. National Library of Medicine lists these common warning signs of significant dehydration:

- Not being able to urinate, or urinating very little

- Urine that is highly concentrated and dark yellow in color

- Not being able to produce tears

- Sunken eyes

- In infants, the soft spot on the head is significantly sunken

- Lethargy, dizziness, or lightheadedness

- Dry mouth

If your body is hydrated, you should be producing colorless urine. Side effects of dehydration can include stress, headaches, back pain, asthma, weight gain, allergies, high blood pressure, and Alzheimer's disease.

What is a healthy amount of water to drink?

The Institute of Medicine advises that men consume roughly 3 liters (about 13 cups) of water a day, and women, 2.2 liters (about 9 cups) per day. You should always be sipping water, and never go more than 15 or 20 minutes without. The very first thing you should do when you get out of bed is have a big glass of water with lemon in it. After a night's sleep is when you are the most dehydrated and toxic. Also, drink water 15 to 20 minutes before a meal to support the digestive process.

Can you overdose on water?

A 2005 study in the New England Journal of Medicine found that close to one-sixth of marathon runners develop some degree of hyponatremia, or dilution of the blood caused by drinking too much water, resulting in very low blood sodium levels. This condition has made many people very sick and even close to death.

In humans, the kidneys control the amount of water, salts, and other solutes leaving the body by filtering blood through their millions of twisted tubules. When a person drinks excessive amounts of water, the kidneys cannot flush it out fast enough, and the blood becomes waterlogged. Drawn to regions where the concentration of salt and other dissolved substances is higher, excess water leaves the blood and ultimately enters the cells, which swell like balloons to accommodate it. This includes moving into the brain cells. The brain cells then have no room to expand. They press against the skull and compress the brain stem, which controls some of our most important functions like breathing. The results can be deadly.

Dr. Batmanghelidj, an expert on the natural healing

power of water, reminds us of the importance of balancing sodium intake with water consumption. He recommends the following: Take ¼ teaspoon of salt per quart (about 4-5 glasses) of water. Make sure you're taking the right kind of salt, NOT table salt. The best form of salt to use is Celtic sea salt or Himalayan sea salt.

Is tap water healthy?

In 2005, the nonprofit Environmental Working Group (EWG) tested municipal water in 42 states and detected some 260 contaminants in public water supplies, 140 of which were unregulated chemicals. In other words, public officials have no safety standards for these chemicals, or any plans for how to remove them.

The bottom line is clean drinking water is a very scarce commodity. It won't be long before the world is fighting over water instead of oil. National statistics do not tell us about the quality and safety of the water that is coming out of our taps. This is because drinking water quality varies from place to place, depending on the source and the treatment it receives. Many of our faucets are drawing polluted water.

Think about this. We have miles and miles of pipes under our streets and homes. Are these pipes securely sealed? Can germs, rust, corrosion, seepage, rats, and all kinds of other hazards get into our tap water before we draw it out of the tap and pour it into the glasses we drink from?

Is bottled water healthy?

Some bottled water is treated more than tap water, and some is treated less or not at all. The Natural Resources Defense Council (NRDC) has researched bottled water extensively, and found that the standards for the treatment and testing of bottled water are not as high as those for tap water. Bottled water is tested less frequently than tap water for bacteria and chemical contaminants. Additionally, the U.S Food and Drug and Administration allows for some contamination by E. coli or fecal contaminants in the water, contrary to the EPA tap water rules, which prohibit any such contamination. This may be a good indication that bottled water may not be the best choice.

Eric Olsen, of the Natural Resources Defense Council, says the realization that bottled water is seldom of higher quality than tap water has caused a major shift in opinion. San Francisco, Los Angles, Phoenix, Chicago, St. Louis, and many other cities have made it illegal to spend city dollars on bottled water.

Powerful reasons not to drink bottled water

All plastic bottles leach synthetic chemicals into water, some more than others. Massive amounts of greenhouse gases are produced from manufacturing plastic bottles. All tallied, 60 million plastic bottles a day are disposed of in America alone! Millions of gallons of fuel are wasted daily transporting filtered tap water across America and around the world. It requires three times as much water to make the bottles as it does to fill them. It is a massive, wasteful industry. Just about every study on bottled water shows contamination from bacteria or synthetic chemicals. Approximately 80 percent of bottled water brands are processed water. This means that municipal or tap water has been run through a filtration system to remove impurities or chemicals. Take, for example, Dasani (from Coke) or Aquafina (from Pepsi). These waters are simply bottled from municipal water supplies. I just can't see any good in promoting the bottled water industry.

What is the best type of water?

Here is a very simple alternative to using bottled water and polluting our world. The best way to have pure water is to eliminate all contaminants that come out of your tap. With the right home water filtration system, you can have complete control over what you drink. To have a great, healthy life, you cannot afford to leave it to chance. This is the most economical, most convenient, and healthiest alternative to tap or bottled water. A home water filtration system will be the most valuable home appliance you own; it will ensure the safety of your drinking water for you and your family. Think of the importance of having healthy, chemical-free water. It literally could save your life. Join the millions of informed consumers who "just say no" to bottled water and tap water. It is healthier for you, for our economy, for your family, and for our planet. All good brands are certified by NSF International, an Ann Arbor, Michigan-based nonprofit standards group. You can now enjoy great-tasting, purified water, and rest easy that the water you are drinking is free of pollutants and cancer-causing toxins.

Extreme nutrition

This program is designed to show you how to get maximum energy – the most powerful resource we have within us to maximize our capacity as human beings. At times, you may notice that your energy is depleted, your body is out of balance, and you are not operating at an optimal level. Keeping your energy up and your body balanced is simple. By maintaining a proper ratio between the acidity and alkalinity in your body, you can re-energize your life.

Basically, the foods you are putting in your body and which foods you are combining together determine if you are going to maintain great health. Being overweight, fatigued, or lethargic are all caused by having too much acid in the body. The typical American diet produces a vast amount of acid in the body. It is impossible to be truly healthy when the body is consistently producing high acid levels.

Dr. Robert O. Young, in his book, The pH Miracle, puts it like this: "Those willing to look again, and with clear eyes, will be rewarded with the secrets to permanent health." We can heal ourselves by changing the environment inside

146

our bodies. Potentially harmful invaders will then have nowhere to grow and will become harmless. The concept of acid/alkaline imbalance as the cause of disease in the body is not a new one. Edgar Cayce was one of the very first to aim to alkalize the body through detoxification with herbs, fasting, colonics, massages, steam baths, and diet modification.

Sam Whang, the author of the book, Reverse Aging, says, "Even if we eat organic fruit and vegetables, 97% of our food still consists of carbon, nitrogen, hydrogen, and oxygen. This will still be reduced to acid waste." He says it is not what we put in our bodies, but what stays in our bodies as waste that creates the condition of being overly acidic, and causes us to age prematurely. In terms of acid/alkaline balance, says Whang, the only difference between good food and bad food is that good food will have less acid waste and more acid neutralizing results. Your pH balance depends on what is left after metabolism.

The smart dieters I know who have created an alkaline balance in their bodies have a better quality of life. You start experiencing massive improvement in health. Your mind becomes stronger, your energy increases, your stamina and strength build, your concentration improves, and your body becomes resistant to diseases. And, of course, you lose weight. Your entire body functions more efficiently, just as it was meant to.

Balance in the body is a very important concept. If we want our bodies to function properly, it comes down to balance. For example, we know that when our muscles work hard, they must get sufficient rest. When you breathe, you must inhale and then exhale. When you consume calories, you must burn them off. In addition, when the body produces toxins, it must be capable of eliminating them.

The way the body works is fascinating. Vitamins, minerals, sugars, fatty acids, amino acids, and various other elements are responsible for guiding the body to grow and function properly. It sounds complex but it is really very basic: Each of these components is designed to fulfill a unique purpose, and as a result of working by themselves or with other components, the body is able to perform all of our daily activities without us asking anything of it. Each one of these components that make up the body can be categorized as either an alkaline (or basic) substance or an acidic substance. The same amount of acids and alkalis is what is meant by the term pH balance.

Acids and alkaline substances are unique because they can oppose and complement each other at the same time. If you want to have a healthy body, you must have a balance of acids and alkalis. If you are eating a nutritionally balanced diet, it is not that difficult to balance the two. When acidity and alkalinity are not balanced in the body, a number of health issues can arise.

At this point, you are probably wondering what pH means. The p stands for potential and the H stands for hydrogen. So then, what is potential hydrogen? It refers to the ability to attract hydrogen ions. In simpler terms, pH means the acid/alkaline balance. The pH scale runs from 0 to 14, with the number 7 being the neutral point. The farther below seven you go, the more acidic you are. The higher above seven, the more alkaline you are.

Anyone consuming a typical American diet will most always be low on the pH scale. Put simply, they have too much acid in their system. For those who find the right balance, weight loss is simple. If you want to lose weight, you just have to increase your alkalinity. When alkaline and acidic foods come together, they can neutralize each other. However, to achieve this effect, they have to come together in certain proportions. It takes about 20 times more alkaline substances in the blood to neutralize a given amount of acid. What this means is you need to take in a lot more alkalizing foods than acidic foods. Once you get to a healthy pH level, it is a lot easier to maintain it than it is to initially get to that healthy pH level from an overly acidic state.

So what actually constitutes a healthy body? Well, mainstream medicine says you should have a reading of about 7.3 to 7.45 for a normal blood pH level. "Normal" is based on the average American; the problem is that the average American is overweight or obese. This means that this range does not reflect the pH level of a healthy person! Dr. Robert Young suggests you should be in the range from 7.350 to 7.380, and the ideal would be 7.365 (slightly alkaline). He considers mainstream medicine's "normal" range to be sufficient for survival, and the ideal range represents great health.

The reason acidosis, the condition of being overly acidic, is so common in our society is largely because of the typical American diet, which is far too high in acid-producing animal products like meat, eggs, and dairy, and far too low in alkali-producing foods like fresh vegetables. Additionally, we eat acid-producing processed foods like white flour and sugar, and drink acid-producing beverages like coffee and soft drinks. We use too many drugs, which are acid-forming, and we use artificial chemical sweeteners like NutraSweet, Equal, or Aspartame, which are extremely acid-forming. One of the best things we can do to correct an overly acidic body is to clean up our diet and lifestyle.

What is acidic?

The majority of people in North America do eat some alkalizing foods, but not nearly enough. A couple of pieces of fruit and a small plate of vegetables alone are not enough to offset the acid formed by the majority of the food consumed. Whether or not a substance is classified as an acid has to do with what happens when the substance dissolves in water. If the substance releases hydrogen ions, it is considered acid. The number of hydrogen ions that are released determines whether a substance is more or less acidic.

One way to identify an acid is by taste. Most of us can automatically classify lemons or soda pop as acidic purely based on how they taste. But you cannot rely solely on the taste of food to determine if it is acidic or not. Meat, for example, does not have an acidic taste, yet it is an extremely acidic food. Some foods that are classified as acids don't taste acidic because they do not release as many hydrogen ions as do other more noticeably acidic foods. And the acidic taste of other foods is lessened due to the fact that acids may be easily neutralized when combined with other foods. Do not let the taste of foods fool you into engaging in choices that will lead to an unhealthy body.

What can the corrosive nature of acid do?

There is a well-known experiment in which a piece of meat and a coin were soaked in a cola-based beverage. After several days, the meat totally dissolved, and the surface of the coin was scarred and pitted.

A surprising number and variety of physical problems and diseases can be caused by foods that are acid-producing after digestion. Today, the vast majority of the populace in industrialized nations suffers from problems caused by acidosis, because modern diets and lifestyles promote acidification of the body's internal environment.

Acidosis causes health problems

It is critically important that your pH level is properly balanced because it affects everything. For example, if your pH is not balanced, your body cannot effectively assimilate vitamins, minerals, and other nutrients. Research shows that the body benefits from a pH level that is slightly alkaline. Acidosis, or excessive levels of acid in the body, will not only decrease the body's ability to absorb nutrients, but also decrease energy production in the cells. As a result, the body cannot properly repair damaged cells or remove heavy metals and other toxins. In an acidic environment, tumor cells thrive, and the body becomes more susceptible to fatigue and illness.

Acidosis can result from an acid-forming diet, emotional stress, toxic overload, immune reactions, or anything that deprives the cells of oxygen and other nutrients. The body will work to compensate for an acidic pH by using alkaline minerals. If the diet does not contain adequate minerals to compensate, then excess acids get stored in your fat cells (which is a major cause of weight gain). And over a period of time, your body will leach calcium and alkaline stores from your bones in a frantic attempt to retain the pH balance in your body (which is why some people get shorter as they get older).

What difference does toxic blood make?

For the body to remain alive and healthy, it must keep a very precisely balanced blood pH of 7.365, which is slightly alkaline. The body will do whatever it takes in order to maintain this balance.

Your blood plays a very important role in your overall health and well-being. It transports oxygen to all your cells, giving you energy and keeping you alive. It also plays a key role in how energizing your sleep is.

When you are in a deep sleep, proper hydration and blood flow are important. When your blood cells are spaced apart from each other, as they appear in the below image, your blood can move effortlessly throughout your entire body, and is able to get into all your small capillaries. So your sleep becomes more energizing, and you need less of it.

Your blood cells have a negative charge on the outside and a positive charge on the inside; that's what keeps them

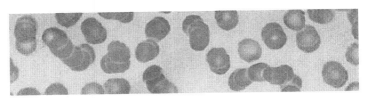

healthy and far apart. When your body is acidic, the acid strips your blood of its negative charge. Your blood cells no longer have the same repelling force; they come together and form big clumps, as shown in the picture below.

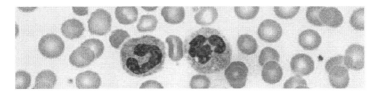

When your blood starts to clump together, it will no longer get through all the little capillaries in your body to deliver the oxygen you need to stay healthy. It will no longer be able to give all of the cells in your body the energizing and rejuvenating effects they need. This is a major cause of why many people feel horrible when they wake up, and need to go back to bed. It's also a big reason why you wake up feeling dehydrated.

I grew up where it was very cold in the winter time, with snow and sometimes minus 40 degree Celsius temperatures, not even taking the wind chill factor into account. Very often I would hear things like, "Dress warmly or you'll catch a cold!" Or, "Don't get your feet wet!" When we are growing up, we often hear warnings like this so we are programmed to think that diseases are all around us, that they're going to get us. "Don't touch the escalator handle; you may get germs!" The truth is, we create a toxic environment inside our body.

Seventy percent of our body is water. And most of the time, because of our diet, emotions, stress and lifestyle, the water in our body is overly acidic. Simply put, it's toxic. Even more scary, modern day medicine puts so much attention on fighting the symptoms, and not recognizing the root cause of problems. In effect, we are paying for drugs that will supposedly make us healthy, but may only contribute to our problems. (This topic will be in my complete health CD course, which you can find on my website.)

What is Alkaline?

When a substance does not give up its hydrogen ions after being placed in a solution of water, it is considered alkaline. Alkaline substances differ from acids in that they are not corrosive; they are much gentler. Calcium, the most prominent mineral inside the body, is an example of an alkaline substance.

Here are some sure ways to help alkalize your body:

1. Reduce your intake of sugar and products made from sugar, including soda pop, pies, ice cream, jello, jams, jellies, artificial juices, puddings, doughnuts, corn syrups, chewing gum, sweetened drinks, cookies, breakfast cereals, liqueurs, and mixed drinks. Preferably, you should eliminate them completely.

2. Avoid processed foods and condiments, including ketchup, salad dressings, pickles, luncheon meats, canned fruits, breads made from refined flour, relish, cheese dips, peanut butter, prepared seafood, frozen vegetables, crackers, canned soups, hot dogs, sausages, and sweetened yogurt.

3. Eliminate cooking and re-heating food and drinks in the microwave.

4. Eliminate dairy, meats, fried foods, and fast foods. There are many great alternatives.

5. Increase your consumption of fresh, raw fruits and vegetables. You should include raw vegetables in every meal. If your breakfast is so small that you only eat toast or cereal, stop eating toast and take fresh fruits or vegetable juices instead. If your lunches usually consist of sandwiches, try to substitute them with a raw salad or a vegetable juice. Have a salad before you eat every meal.

This way, you will be sure to eat all of the salad instead of finding yourself too full to finish it.

6. Include more whole grains. Grains form the base of a balanced diet, and are important in maintaining the alkaline balance in the body. Grains are a great source of vitamins, minerals, and essential nutrients, including folic acid, fiber, carbohydrates, antioxidants, and phyto-estrogens. The Department of Food Science and Nutrition at the University of Minnesota determined that consumption of whole grains reduces the risk of chronic diseases, including cancer and cardiovascular disease. By eating grains, you can eat less, but still feel full. Grains should comprise about 20% of your diet.

Alkalinity for cancer prevention

Have you ever thought about why the heart never gets cancer? The truth is, the heart will never get this disease. Cancer is not compatible with a healthy pH environment full of oxygen.

An alkaline diet is perhaps one of the only known ways to help prevent cancer. Let me briefly explain what causes cancer, and why an alkaline diet will help with prevention. All of our cells take in oxygen, nutrients, and glucose, while they get rid of toxins. The immune system protects the cells. As soon as the body starts to get acidic, the immune system is affected by the toxins, and cells lose their capacity to keep taking in oxygen, and thus ferment. The question is, if you create a body that is more alkaline than acid, can that help prevent cancer?

Cancer cells sit dormant at a pH of 7.4, and as the body ups its alkalinity and the pH level reaches 8.4, these malignant cells die off. So, yes, the more alkaline you are, the better chance you have to fight off this disease. Cancer cells are anaerobic, and can only live in very low oxygen conditions. Because cancer cannot live in an oxygenated environment, the more oxygen the cells have, the better the chance to prevent cancer. Alkaline tissue can hold up to twenty times more oxygen than acidic tissue. So the more acidic tissues the body has, the more likely it will be a fertile ground for cancer to grow and spread. When a person consumes an alkaline diet, this helps the cells get enough oxygen and discard their toxic wastes. Cancer will not take hold under circumstances like this. So to beat cancer, make sure you have a lot of alkalizing foods in your diet. Examples of alkalizing foods include:

- Vegetables: especially raw, green, leafy vegetables.

- Fresh herbs and spices: parsley, basil, cilantro, cayenne, ginger.

- Fruits: watermelon, avocado, cucumber, young coconuts.

- Wheat grass.

- Sprouts, such as: alfalfa, bean, broccoli.

How to Test Your Body's Acidity or Alkalinity using pH Strips

I highly suggest that you test your pH levels to determine if your body's pH balance needs immediate attention. By using pH test strips, you can determine your pH factor very quickly in the privacy of your own home. The best time to test your pH is about one hour before a meal or two hours after a meal. I check my pH levels twice per month. You can pick up the strips in any health food store, drug store, or on the Internet.

Acidosis, an extended time in the acid pH state, can result in rheumatoid arthritis, diabetes, lupus, tuberculosis, osteoporosis, high blood pressure, cancers, and many more diseases. If your salivary pH stays too low, your diet should focus on fruit, vegetables and, mineral water, and you should remove strong acidifiers such as sodas and red meat.

Things we should never put in our body

Fructose

In the 1960s, Americans went from consuming no fructose to eating more than 63 pounds of it every year. Fructose is a major reason we are so overweight. Many foods, even some labeled as low fat, have fructose in them. Fructose does not turn off hunger signals, and you will just keep eating and eating.

Avoid foods with any of these ingredients listed in the top five on a food label: high fructose corn syrup, and enriched, bleached, or refined flour. These ingredients are simple, refined sugars with few nutrients left. The only way to prevent yourself from eating these ingredients that could literally kill you over time is to start reading every label before you buy.

Sweeteners

One of the leading causes of inflammation is sucrose (sugar). You can decrease this effect by using alternative sweeteners. Agave nectar is a natural substance, and one of the healthiest sugar substitutes available; however, it is higher in calories. You only have to use half the amount of agave nectar as you would sugar for the same amount of sweetness.

Saturated fats versus unsaturated fats

All fats have the same number of calories, but they are not all created equal. A diet high in foods that contain unsaturated fats instead of saturated fats can help reduce your blood cholesterol level.

Monosodium glutamate (MSG)

We have all most likely had Chinese food and other foods containing monosodium glutamate (MSG), a sodium salt. MSG can play a major role in upsetting your metabolism. This additive basically enhances the taste of food. But what it also does is overstimulate the glutamine receptors of the brain, so we crave salt and sweets more. This can cause us to eat more and to have higher insulin levels. I could go on about MSG and its harmful effects, but the bottom line is, don't eat it if you want to experience a long healthy life.

Fats that will kill you

Did you know that trans fats were originally made from candle wax? So how healthy do you think they can be for us. Saturated fats and trans fats will kill us over time. These are the number one foods that will clog your arteries and kill you, and they are the number one foods that lead to weight gain. Think about bad fats as being solid at room temperature, foods such as butter, stick margarine, lard, and animal fats. Foods containing trans fats have a very long shelf life, and that puts more money into the pockets of food manufacturers. Trans fats consist of hydrogenated vegetable oil, which is the worst kind of fat you can put in your system. They will stop all your weight loss efforts dead in their tracks.

What alcohol really does

Many of us think we should not drink alcohol because of the calories consumed. That is only a tiny portion of why alcohol contributes to weight gain. A big reason is that alcohol lowers your inhibition, so when you see junk food, you feel like it is all right to eat it, along with anything else in sight. Then the next day you think, "Why did I eat all that food?"

A major cause of obesity

In today's world, we consume more sugar than ever. In the 1700s, we consumed 7.5 pounds of sugar per capita annually, and today we consume a whopping 150 pounds.

Too many carbohydrates can make you hungry

If you follow an eating plan that is too high in carbs, it can actually make you feel hungry. Limit your carbs to less than 50 percent of your diet. Also, it's important to make sure most of your carbs are complex, foods such as whole grains and vegetables. Always have energy foods ready for hungry cravings. You can turn to things like V8 juice, a handful of nuts, already prepared vegetables, or pieces of fruit. In the food section, I provide you with a list of energy foods.

Protein misconception

I probably have more muscle than most of you reading this book right now, and I'll bet I don't eat nearly as much protein as 95 percent of you. So how can I have so much more muscle tissue than you?

Let me explain. You should actually be more concerned about eating too much protein than not enough. The average American woman eats 144 percent more protein than her recommended daily allowance. The average American man eats 175 percent more than his recommended daily allowance. All the amino acids that your body needs to make complete proteins can be found in plant sources. The healthier your blood is, the more muscle you will build. And the way you create healthier blood is by eating electron-rich green food and good fats, not protein. Gorillas, elephants, and horses are some of the strongest animals in the world and they are not meat eaters but plant eaters. We have been taught that the more protein we eat, the healthier we are; if you don't get enough protein, your bones are going to break. Protein is essential for building muscle. But too much of it decreases appetite and, therefore, we miss meals and the fat starts to build up. To meet your daily protein requirements, you need only two ounces per day.

What will happen to me if I cut out dairy?

We often drink more milk to beat osteoporosis, and yet in the United States, England, and Sweden, we have the highest rates of osteoporosis in the world and drink the most milk. Think about all the dairy you get from cheese, ice cream, yogurt, and milk. The average American woman consumes two pounds of milk per day for her whole life, and yet 30 million have osteoporosis.

Drinking more milk will not prevent bone loss. In fact, taking in too much protein can cause bone loss. Science magazine in 1986 called dietary protein the most important contributor to osteoporosis. In 1995, the American Journal of Clinical Nutrition said protein increases production of acid in the blood, which can be neutralized by calcium mobilized from the skeleton. In 1991, the American Journal of Clinical Nutrition found that even someone getting 1,400 milligrams of calcium daily can lose up to 4 percent of their bone mass each year on a high protein diet. Vast research was done on the effects of dairy intake on the bones at Harvard, Yale, and Penn State. Not one of those studies found that dairy will help prevent osteoporosis. A more interesting study done by the National Dairy Council found that the high protein content of dairy actually leaches calcium from the body. Why do they not have a commercial exposing that information? Because they're a multi-billion dollar industry, motivated by money. It's not hard to figure out that we need to reduce the excess protein in our diets so our body will not leach calcium from the bones to neutralize metabolic acids, and weaken them.

Many dairy products also have concentrated sugars called lactose. Lactose breaks down in the body to lactic acid, which is a big reason we get inflammation and irritation in the bones, joints, and muscles. Mammals need an enzyme called lactase to digest the sugar, lactose. We lose 90 to 95 percent of these enzymes from the age of 18 months to 4 years. Pasteurized milk, which has a lot of acid, and the undigested lactose, cause the growth of bacteria in our intestines. Because cancer cells can live in an acidic environment, this is where we have a greater chance of developing this disease. In addition to colon cancer, a high intake of dairy products has also been associated with an increased risk of breast cancer.

A cow's milk helps a calf grow from 90 pounds to 2,000 pounds in two years. They will double their weight in just 47 days. Do you think that a cow's body works the same way as a human body? Not a chance. Cow's milk is a lot more fattening than human milk; that is why the calf grows so big.

Have you ever noticed that after you have had certain dairy products you start to produce mucus? All dairy products will produce mucus in the body, and we start to develop allergies and colds that work to fight off the attack.

We're the only species on the planet that drinks the milk of another species, and that drinks milk as adults. Why don't we drink other species' milk? Why just cows? I always get a big kick out of people who try to argue with me that milk is good for us. Think about why we choose the cow. It's greatly beneficial to use the animal that will produce the largest amounts of milk, in order to put profits in people's pockets. It has nothing to do with health. The dairy industry has some of the best marketing in the world. It's a multi-billion dollar industry, and money flies in every direction from people who take a piece of the pie, from doctors to the government.

A friend of mine, who is one of the most educated people I know in the area of nutrition, states it like this: "If you want to be sick, keep taking in dairy." You know what makes me sick? Nutritionists and dietitians that say dairy is good for you. Many of them use their expertise to get people to believe information, but they have not stayed up-to-date with new findings in their field.

Do a lot of professionals in the medical field agree that dairy is not great? Yes, so how does the dairy industry get away with spending billions on advertising to market their products? If you sit down at night and watch TV, you will see commercial after commercial, but spend just an hour reading a medical journal, and you will get a different story. Who are you going to believe?

Here is a very important fact you must understand about doctors. Most doctors are not trained in nutrition, and many know nothing about nutrition at all. According to state investigations, doctors receive less than three hours of nutritional training in medical school. This is why a lot of times when an overweight person goes to a doctor, the doctor doesn't deal with the patient's weight problem because they just don't know how. The patients may be depressed because they are overweight, so they give them drugs to help with depression rather than sitting down and creating a plan for how to get into good physical shape.

Let's suppose you still don't believe anything I have told you, and still believe that milk is good for you. Maybe the truth about factory farms will convince you. Under normal circumstances a cow's udders supply about 10 pounds of milk per day. Money hungry farmers inject their cows with a growth hormone called bovine somatotropin that increases milk production to 100 pounds per day.

Here is the truth. At one time in my life, I drank a lot of milk, and I even worked on a dairy farm. Yes, you heard that correctly. I worked on a dairy farm, and also in a meat packing plant. Yes, a slaughter house.

Let me share a quick story with you. When I used to milk cows, I would have to put big metal suction cups on the udders of the cow for milking. Before we put the machine on the udders to milk, we would clean the udders. However, there would be so much feces, bacteria, and contaminants that we could not get it all off. We were on a schedule, and had to get the cows in and out as fast as possible.

Often the udders became infected, but the machines kept milking, sucking the dead white blood cells into the milk. So to get rid of all this, milk must be pasteurized. Pasteurization destroys all the beneficial enzymes and, as a result, less calcium is available, but it does not kill all the viruses or bacteria. Additionally, radioactive particles are found in milk. One hundred percent of cheese products produced and sold in the US have detectable pesticide residues. And dioxin, one of the most toxic substances in the world, is also often found in dairy products.

There is also a protein in cow's milk called casein. There is 300 times more casein in cow's milk than in human milk. That is why cows develop such huge bones. In the stomach, casein starts to coagulate and form large, tough, dense and difficult to digest curds, which is fine for the cow. In our system, the body has to work really hard to get rid of the curds, and uses a massive amount of energy. This blob of substance hardens and adheres to the lining of the intestines, which in turn prevents the absorption of nutrients into the body, resulting in lethargy. The next time you wash your car, spray paint a few lines of milk on it, and see how hard it is to wash off. Dairy products can do the same to your insides. This will actually promote weight gain instead of weight loss. Casein is also the base of one of the strongest glues used in woodworking.

Sugar: good or bad?

Sugar is extremely acidic in the body and is a major cause of obesity. Americans consume 50,000 pounds of sugar weekly. Some sugars to watch out for are white sugar, honey, maple syrup, brown sugar, molasses and corn syrup.

Simple carbs will form in the body from foods such as white flour, white rice, and certain pastas. A lot of these foods can increase your blood sugar. Read all labels for sugars, especially packaged foods. You will be surprised how many sugars are in them.

Artificial sweeteners

Most artificial sweeteners are terrible for you, and are a great way to introduce disease into the body. Aspartame (NutraSweet), saccharin, (Sweet 'n Low), and sucralose (Splenda), for example, all start to cause hazardous acids in your body.

Here is how great aspartame is for you. There is an ingredient in aspartame called methyl alcohol, which converts to formaldehyde, a neurotoxin well known as a carcinogen. In the next stage, it turns into formic acid, the same stuff fire ants use in their attacks. This is just one ingredient in one of the artificial sweeteners. Moreover, these sweeteners cause us to gain weight because the aspartic acid in them is very close to the glutamic acid found in monosodium glutamate (MSG), which promotes weight gain.

Peanuts: healthy or not?

We have heard it for years. Peanuts are not good for our health. Peanuts are very high in acid and contain over 27 yeasts and molds. Peanut butter is a walking death trap. Switch to almond butter; it tastes better and is a lot healthier for you.

Fermented and malted foods

The list of fermented and malted foods includes things like soy sauce, vinegar, miso, tamari, tempeh, olives, and pickles. It also includes many well-known condiments, including ketchup, mustard, mayonnaise, steak sauce, pre-packed salad dressings, relish, and chili sauce. All these condiments are acidic in the body and fermented by fungus.

Alcohol

Alcohol has a pH level of 4.5 and wine coolers have a pH of 2.84, and they are fermented and acidic. Yes, alcohol will make you fat. It also has a lot of bacteria and yeast from the way it is made. The liver can convert alcohol into another very toxic waste product called acetaldehyde. If you must drink alcohol, please do so in very low doses.

Caffeine

I worry when people say to me, "I could never give up coffee," and then they develop some kind of disease in their body, and are told to give it up, but sometimes it's too late. Research has shown that cancer cells can live indefinitely in coffee. Coffee is highly acidic, and if you add cream and sugar, it is outright deadly. If you must drink coffee, I highly suggest you go with black as the pH level is a little better at 5.09, and decaf has an even better pH at 5.22, but acid is acid, so be cautious.

If you have read the chapter about emotional states, you will recall that we only drink coffee to change our state. If it did not give you a quick pick-me-up, you would not drink it. There are many ways to change your state and get energy rather than turning to coffee. If you were to inject one milligram of caffeine into your bloodstream, it could kill you. There is enough in just one ounce of milk chocolate to get rid of six people. Now when it comes to coffee, a strong cup can get rid of 200 people. One of my clients, who owns a very large coffee business that operates all over the world and is worth millions, won't even touch coffee.

Soft drinks

Deadly, deadly, deadly. Drink them and it could be deadly. Do I need to say more? Simply put, they are loaded with sugars and other sweeteners. Some are caffeinated and some are without caffeine, but they are still terrible for you because of the acidity. Soda is saturated with protons, with a pH of about 3.0 – ten thousand times more acidic than distilled water. Sports drinks? Also deadly, and more acidic than beer. Gatorade lemon lime has a pH of 2.95.

A main ingredient in colas is phosphoric acid, and it has a pH of 2.5. That will destroy a nail in four days, completely gone. Phosphoric acid leaches calcium from your bones, making it a leading cause of the increase in osteoporosis. Forty-six percent of children from the ages of 6 to 11 now drink a can of soda per day. We are filling our children with acid, and setting them up on a very quick route to disease. These kids may not know the difference yet, but each person reading this book now does. Americans drink 44 gallons of soft drinks each year, an increase of 131 percent since the 1970s. Soda water or seltzer still contains carbonic acid, and has a pH of about 2.5 – fifty thousand times more acidic than distilled water, and Americans drink about four times as much soda water. Hydrating with good alkaline water is extremely important.

What you don't know about meat could kill you

A recent scientific study from China showed, without any doubt, that people who eat the most animal protein have the most heart disease, cancer, and diabetes. It was proven the diets that are vegetable-based show no such increases in these ailments.

Many people know that pasta prompts a release of insulin, but an even bigger release of insulin is caused by meat. Because we, as humans, cannot fully digest meat as it moves through our system, it damages the intestinal villi. In return, this causes poor blood production and then poor cell production. Remember that we're only as healthy as our cells.

Another problem I have with animal foods is the concept of eating something that has been shot and killed. It is not good for you. Simply put, it is just dead. Why choose to put a dead animal in your system over healing and energizing live plant enzymes?

Humans are not designed to be carnivores; we're designed for the consumption of stable plant food. We do not have the jaws and teeth of a lion to tear apart flesh, nor do we have the short, simple bowels of meat eaters, designed for fast absorption. We have long and complicated digestive tracts.

The American Cancer Society conducted a study over a 10-year period with around 80,000 people focused on losing weight. Some people who ate meat three times per week gained a lot more weight than the people who avoided meat and ate more vegetables. When it comes to meat, you must remember that animals that eat meat can quickly pass it through their digestive systems. However, when we eat meat, it sits in us rotting, decomposing, and fermenting in the colon.

Why do you see meats hanging in a butcher shop? Because the meat has to get to the final desired texture and taste suitable to eat, and it is yeast that causes the aging of the meat. Any meat that is properly prepared for human consumption has to be partially fermented, and because of this, the meat is permeated with acids and acid-generating microforms. Red meat has been linked to so many types of cancer: colon, prostate, and breast cancers, just to name a few.

Pork is even worse. A pig has no lymphatic system to move all the acid out of its body. The metabolic acids are stored in their tissues. That yummy bacon you ate? You might as well just ingest straight acid. Pork very often has high levels of contamination by bacteria, yeast, fungi, and associated waste products and acid. The pigs are often fed grain that is stored for long periods of time in silos and become contaminated with fungi. And most slaughterhouses are not able to fight off further contamination. Some people think that if you cook meat, then it is safe, but most of the mycotoxins in the meat can survive being heated.

Chicken and turkeys are even worse. Large intakes of poultry have been directly linked to colon cancer. The Consumers Union – the advocacy group behind Consumer Reports – reports that there is a 42 percent chance of contamination by Campylobacter jejuni, and a 12 percent chance of contamination by salmonella enteritidis. USDA research confirms this as well. The former is bacteria found in animal feces, the latter in the intestines of farm animals. Both of these bacteria are zoonotic, that is, the illnesses they cause can be transferred from animal to human.

Eggs, on the other hand, contain over 37,500,000 pathological microforms. Just from having one egg alone, you will notice increased bacteria and yeast in the blood within 15 minutes, and it will take the white blood cells up to 72 hours to take care of the contaminants. Even eating one egg per day has been proven to be associated with an increase in colon cancer.

According to former USDA microbiologist, Gerald Kuester, "With the advent of modern slaughter technologies, there are about 50 points during processing where cross-contamination can occur." At the end of the line, the birds are no cleaner than if they had been dipped in a toilet." Studies from the Agriculture Department show that 99 percent of broiler carcasses have detectable levels of E.coli and 30 percent of chickens found on the typical American plate are tainted with salmonella.

Disheartening facts

Most chickens are filled with growth hormones and receive only artificial light, so they often outgrow their bones, leading to fractured legs. Egg laying hens are packed so tight into the cages that their feet actually grow around the wire mesh floors. The small cages cause chickens to fight and peck at each other, and peck the factory farm workers, so they sear their beaks off using a hot knife. When chickens are slaughtered, they are forced into a tiny box that should only hold one chicken, but three or more are crammed in so they are unable to stand or spread their wings.

Pigs and cows are put in such small pens, they can't even turn around. They live in their own urine, feces, vomit, and filth, and have sores and wounds.

Just about half of all antibiotics made in the United States go to farm animals. This causes antibiotic resistance in the people who choose to eat them. A study at the University of California Berkeley linked eating beef to urinary tract infections in women.

What creates the taste in beef and chicken? The urine, otherwise known as uric acid, is what gives the taste to the meat. Uric acid can cause arthritic pain in the body and is highly toxic.

What makes the meat chewable? The meat is tenderized by the putrefactive germs, which come from the colon, and softens the tissues to allow for consumption once the animal has been killed. If, by now, you cannot see why meat is not healthy for us, then I don't know what else to say other than, maybe, good luck.

Look at it this way. It's a lot less expensive to clean up your diet a little and start eating healthier than it is to pay for all the medications when you get sick, and all the other fees for other ailments that result.

Antioxidants

The wide range of colors of fruits and vegetables – the reds, greens, oranges, yellows, and purples come from a variety of chemicals called antioxidants. The important thing about antioxidants is that they help to fight off free radicals.

We actually produce very low levels of free radicals throughout our lifetime, but as we are exposed to the sun, certain pollutants, and of course, poor nutrients that we put into our bodies, this creates an environment for unwanted free radical damage. Free radicals are one of the nastiest things you can have in your system, and very often, they cause the tissue to become rigid and limited in function. Think of it like old age. As you grow older, your body becomes creaky and stiff. This is what aging really is. The uncontrolled free radical damage can play a major role in the hardening of the arteries, cancer, cataracts, arthritis, and many other ailments that develop with age.

However, here is the most important part: We do not naturally have anything to protect us from these free radicals. If we were a plant, it would be a different story. We would have photosynthesis, and produce our own antioxidants. Lucky for us, those antioxidants in plants will work the same way in our bodies. We borrow the antioxidants from plants so we can live a long, healthy life, and fight off all those free radicals that are working so hard to give us a life of misery.

Let me talk about some of the foods you must start incorporating into your healthy eating plan and why they are so important. Some you will find in your local grocery stores, others will be in health food stores and, for sure, others will be in your larger grocery chains. All in all, there will be choices for everyone.

Nuts

Many of us have a misconception about nuts and calorie intake. The great thing about nuts is that only 5 to 15 percent of the calories from nuts are not absorbed by the intestinal system. This high absorption rate is a result of how we chew the nuts and how the skins of the nuts influence digestion. Calories are very slowly released throughout the intestinal system, which in return leads to the state of feeling satiated. Not all nuts are created equal. I am speaking specifically about walnuts, almonds, cashews, pecans, and Brazil nuts.

The importance of leafy greens

Leafy greens are a rich source of chlorophyll, a very important ingredient to provide more alkalinity for your body and get rid of stress. Chlorophyll even does something more important; it oxygenates your blood and cleanses it. I add chlorophyll to my water every day. There is an abundance of live enzymes in raw chlorophyll-containing plants. These help enhance the rejuvenation of our cells. If you want to have a biologically younger-looking body, incorporate leafy green vegetables with exercise.

You really can't go wrong with any kind of leafy green vegetables. Let me give you some of my favorites: mustard greens, swiss chard, spinach, romaine lettuce, red leaf lettuce, dinosaur kale, dandelion greens, collards, butter lettuce, beet greens, and arugula.

Vegetables high in fiber

Green beans, green peas, zucchini, sugar snap peas, onions, daikon, cucumbers, celery ,carrots, bok choy, beets, asparagus, green and red peppers, eggplant, asparagus, turnips, and artichokes are all excellent sources of fiber.

Sea vegetables, the most nutritious foods in the world

Listen closely to this fact. Sea vegetables have about 10 times the calcium as cow's milk, and a lot more iron than red meat. They are very alkaline in the system, loaded with chlorophyll, and very digestible. They are also a rich source of naturally-occurring electrolytes, which give us more endurance throughout our day and help us stay hydrated longer.

My favorite sea vegetables:

Kelp and dulse are the most popular known sea vegetables in our culture. Other sea vegetables are kombu, agar, arame and wakame.

Legumes

You must start making legumes part of your daily eating habits. They are high in protein, fiber, vitamins, and minerals. Lentils and split peas are the two legumes I use the most due to their convenience. Gradually increase your consumption each day so your digestive system can adapt. You can now even find vegetarian pea protein concentrates and isolates. If you have soy allergies, this is a good choice. Legumes are great for sprouting, which leaves more of the nutritional value intact. Not a necessity, but a healthier choice.

My favorite legumes:

Lentils- brown, green, and red

Peas- green (split), yellow (split), black-eyed

Beans- black, adzuki, garbanzo (chickpeas), fava, kidney, navy, and pinto

Flaxseeds

Of all the plants, flaxseeds have the highest level of omega-3 essential fatty acids. The body cannot produce omega-3 and omega-6, so these are considered essential. Flaxseed contains a lot of omega-3 and omega-6. Ground whole flaxseed is important in the fat burning process, and just one tablespoon will help the body burn fat as fuel. Omega-3 will also help reduce inflammation caused by movement.

A person who is training, and feeds their muscles with only carbohydrates will store only enough glycogen to last about a 90-minute workout. A person who is training, and includes omega-3 and omega-6 in their diet will draw upon fat reserves, which means this person has a dual force and it will take longer before all glycogen is depleted. This person will be able to perform a lot longer and create a leaner body.

When our body sweats, we lose potassium. Flaxseeds are very high in potassium, and can keep our body stocked with the right amount. Potassium also regulates fluid balance, and will help our body stay hydrated.

You always hear it said: "To lose weight, eat more fiber." Well, flaxseeds contain soluble fiber. This helps slow the release of carbohydrates into the bloodstream and, as a result, helps control insulin and give you more energy. This is why you have to eat fiber; soluble fiber gives the body a sense of feeling full, directing your hungry signal to turn off. If you want to lose weight, increase your intake of fiber.

Flaxseed, like hemp, also has anti-inflammatory properties. When purchasing flaxseed, choose whole flaxseed rather than flaxseed meal. The flaxseed meal is nothing but the oils that have been extracted from the whole flaxseed. You will see flaxseed meal used as a filler in baked goods or low-end meal replacements. Whole flax seed has all the nutrients still intact. A good way to get the best nutrients out of your whole seeds is to grind them up in your coffee grinder. This will expose all their oils and nutritional value so they can be used very effectively by the body. Grind them and store in an air-tight container in the refrigerator for up to three months. Flaxseeds are small with very hard shells, and can easily pass through the system undigested when consumed whole. That's why I recommend grinding them for complete nutrition.

Hemp

This is where I learned one of my first big lessons on health. At one time in my life, I used to body build, so I took in tons of proteins, which at the time, I thought was healthy for me. I looked great on the outside, but was harming myself on the inside. I have lost two friends with whom I used to body build. Now I look back and realize that they both developed cancer in their 30s and died due to the type and amount of protein in their diets, which played a large part in them getting sick. It is too bad I was not more educated in the area of health back then.

I started consuming my protein as hemp protein. Most of the mainstream proteins on the shelves in the health food store are acidic in your body. Hemp has really started to hit the mainstream now and people are starting to understand the extreme health benefits. Hemp is a whole food in its natural state so you don't have to create isolates or extracts from it.

In the health food stores, you will see a lot of protein isolates. Hemp protein contains all 10 essential amino acids and has a higher pH level than any other protein. We must obtain essential amino acids through diet because the body does not produce them. The strong amino acid mix will speed up recovery and boost the body's immune system. Moreover, when we perform physical activity, we break down tissues, and because hemp has anti-inflammatory properties, it will speed up your recovery. Edestin is an amino acid that you will only find in hemp, and is a big part of your DNA. This is what makes the hemp plant closest to our own amino acid profile.

Because hemp is totally raw, the digestive enzymes remain the same, allowing the body to take it in with ease, cutting down on digestive strain. Basically, you will be able digest this protein so much easier than other proteins. I even started to save money with hemp protein, because when you buy a good quality protein you don't have to take nearly as much.

This protein is important because it will release the hormones that help the body utilize its fat reserves, which will help you lose more weight and give you more endurance.

The most important thing is that hemp is kept in its raw state. It does not lose its high-end balanced fats, vitamins, minerals, antioxidants, fiber, or the alkaline chlorophyll. When you are buying hemp food – including hemp seed, hemp oil, and my favorite, hemp protein powder – you need to make sure it's fresh. Look for hemp that has been grown with no herbicides or pesticides. It should have a pleasant smell and be very green in color and taste, like the farmer just harvested it.

Pumpkin seeds

Pumpkin seeds are extremely important if you don't eat a lot of meat. I snack on pumpkin seeds all the time. They are very rich in iron. Keep pumpkin seeds around the house to sprinkle on your meals.

Anemia – a shortage of red blood cells in the body – is usually caused by low iron or strenuous exercise. When you exercise, you start to lose iron because the blood cells get crushed due to muscle contractions, and the more you exercise the more iron you need. Iron can also be lost through sweets. Bottom line, you should exercise for the rest of your life, so that means you will need more iron. Keep pumpkin seeds around at all times.

Sesame seeds

You want to get more calcium, but not through milk. Instead, start taking in more sesame seeds, which are high in calcium and extremely absorbable. It's true that if you want strong bones and teeth, you need more calcium. It seems crazy to me how much money has been put into milk commercials since I was young to program us into believing that milk is the best way to get calcium.

If you live in a warm climate, you need extra calcium due to loss from sweating. A good thing to do is to grind the sesame seeds up in your coffee maker, store the seeds in your fridge for up to three months, and sprinkle them on any meals you like. Don't you think this is a great way to keep your kids healthy? And you can finally start using your coffee grinder for something healthy.

Sunflower seeds

You should be eating sunflower seeds on a regular basis. They contain 22 percent protein, and several vitamins that you need for good health. They are also high in trace minerals, vitamin E, and are antioxidant rich.

Pseudo-grains

Pseudo-grains are some of my favorites and I eat them often. They are very alkaline in the system and could be in a category by themselves. These are actually seeds, yet most people think they're grains. One of the reasons why they are called grains is because they can substitute nicely as a grain. They contain no gluten, making them very easily digestible. On a nutritional level, these seeds stand way above any other foods.

Here are some of the choices I like the best and their nutritional value:

Buckwheat

As I state in your eating plan, buckwheat is great to have as a cereal in your most important meal of the day, breakfast. It is rich in the essential amino acid, tryptophan, an important component in the making of serotonin.

You will notice a change in your mood – no more mood swings – and you will have more mental clarity. It is very high in protein, and recently there have been studies done on its powerful ability to bind cholesterol. There are also studies being done for the treatment of high blood pressure, elevated cholesterol, and type 2 diabetes. Additionally, it is a great source of vitamins B and E, and manganese. That's a great start for your morning breakfast.

Amaranth

When people tell me you can only get your calcium from cow's milk, I often laugh. Amaranth has two times the calcium milk does; it has five times the iron of wheat flour, and three times the fiber. It is also high in potassium, phosphorous, and vitamins A, K and E. This is literally a super food. It is a calcium-delivering powerhouse that is rich in lysine, a unique essential amino acid not found in many plant sources. What lysine does is assist your body in absorbing calcium in the digestive tract. If you're looking for a highly digestible food, this one is 90 percent digestible.

Quinoa

I eat quinoa on a regular basis, quite often a quinoa salad from my local grocery store for lunch. Out of all of the pseudo-grains, quinoa is the highest in protein, with 20 percent. It has lots of iron and potassium. It also has a lot of lysine in it.

Wild rice

Wild rice is another food I love to eat often. It also is packed with lysine, high in B vitamins, and it grows in my own backyard on the Canadian prairies. It is very seldom treated with pesticides, making it that much healthier. It is an aquatic grass that originated in North America, and grows best in the wild.

Extra virgin olive oil

Extra virgin means the oil is from the first pressing of the olive. This is a very healthy choice, good in taste and color, and can be used in sauces, dips and dressings, but it only offers a small amount of omega-3.

Hemp oil

Hemp oil is one the healthiest oils on the market. You have already heard me rave about how good hemp is. Each and every one of you should have products in your pantry that say hemp. Hemp oil is made by pressing the hemp seed. It's a dark green color, and has a very soft, smooth texture. I love to use this on my salads as dressing. It is unique because of its ideal ratio of omega-6 and omega-3 fatty acids.

Pumpkin seed oil

Pumpkin seed oil has a large amount of essential fatty acids, and many studies show it has helped improve prostate health. This is a must for men, as the leading cancer for men is prostate cancer.

Almonds

Almonds are one of the best nuts in my books by far. Take a handful 20 minutes before you eat, and they will help you eat a lot less. They are high in vitamin B13, fiber, and antioxidants, and have one of the highest nutrient values of all the nut family. You can also soak your nuts to make them more nutritious but you don't have to. They can be soaked and kept in the fridge for up to one week. They will help you feel fuller longer so you don't eat as much.

Grains

Here is a list of my favorite grains and the ones that are the healthiest:

Whole Grain Brown rice

We can all easily make the change to brown rice. It used to be that all sushi was made with white rice; now, many places are starting to make sushi with brown rice as well. It goes to show that brown rice is finally starting to catch on in the mainstream. It is about time.

What makes brown rice different from white is the processing of the rice. The processing of brown rice is very simple, keeping a lot of the rice in its natural state. The outermost layer, the hull, is retained, so the rice retains most of its nutrient value. It is incredibly high in manganese, and has large amounts of selenium and magnesium. It is also a good source of vitamin B.

If you get tired of brown rice, substitute Thai black rice or purple sticky rice at a 1:1 ratio. If you want to add more flavor to the rice, when cooking, add 1 teaspoon of rooibos leaves for each uncooked cup of rice.

Millet

Millet is gluten-free, and becomes slightly alkaline in the body. Millet can be either creamy or fluffy, depending on how you cook it, and is the most easily digestible of all the grains. Millet is great because it can go with many meals. It's high in vitamin B, magnesium, and the essential amino acid tryptophan, and is nutritionally dense. Millet flour can be used in a wide range of recipes as well.

Spelt

I like spelt, and have some type of spelt salad every day. What I like about spelt is that is has not been tampered with over time. That is why we call spelt an ancient grain, with its long, healthy history. Spelt has 30 percent more protein and less gluten than your average whole wheat. Spelt works well with other grain and seed flours for baking.

Teff

Teff is an intriguing grain, ancient, minute in size, and packed with nutrition. Teff is believed to have originated in Ethiopia between 4,000 and 1,000 BC. Teff seeds were discovered in a pyramid thought to date back to 3,359

BC. The grain has been widely r
countries, including Ethiopia, '
Australia. Teff is known as a c
it is ground into flour, ferme
made into injera, a sourdour
used as porridge and as ⌐
alcoholic drinks. Teff is not wiu⌐
U.S., although it is cultivated in Souⅼı.
and is available in many health food stores.

Teff grains are so small that the majority of the ɥ.
consists of the bran and germ. This makes it very nutrient
dense because the germ and bran are the most nutritious
parts of the grain. The grain also has a very high calcium
content, and contains high levels of phosphorous, iron,
copper, aluminum, barium, and thiamin. It is has one of
the best amino acid compositions, with lysine levels higher
than wheat or barley. It has a lot of protein, carbohydrates,
and fiber. Teff also has no gluten in it. Teff becomes creamy
when cooked; if you want a crunchy texture, reduce the
cooking time.

Chlorella

This is by far one of the most powerful super foods on
the planet and an absolute must for you. Chlorella contains
more chlorophyll than any other plant.

And you must understand by now that chlorophyll will
literally help you live a longer, healthier life. Chlorella is the
fastest growing plant in the world. It is a nutritious, fresh
water green algae, and is one of the very few plants that
produce vitamin B12.

This plant is very strongly alkalizing and well received
in the vegan world. People always ask, where do you get
protein if you don't eat meat? Well, chlorella contains 65
percent protein and possesses 19 amino acids, including
ten essentials, not to mention all the fatty acids, the vitamins, minerals, and enzymes. Chlorella will even enhance
the efficiency of the immune system at the cellular level.

st get into the habit of taking chlorella daily.
mportant. The reason I take chlorella daily is it
p cell regeneration and muscle recovery, enhances
, and slows aging. It will also help you when you are
nd stressed by supporting your immune system, and
elps with cell repair.

Chlorella growth factor (CGF) is a compound that plays a major role in chlorella. It is responsible for causing chlorella to quadruple every day, and we can greatly benefit from its growth factor. CGF is what helps the body's immune system fight off stress, disease, and sickness. Chlorella will help fight off the cellular damage caused by nasty free radicals produced by vehicle emissions.

To choose the best chlorella, look for brands with high protein and chlorophyll content. Read the labels. Look for 65 to 70 percent protein, and 6 to 7 percent chlorophyll. Many people ask me, can you take too much of this? The answer is, no. I recommend taking about 1 teaspoon daily. I take up to 1 tablespoon when I am training a lot. I notice a difference in my recovery time and overall feeling of well-being. Chlorella does contain iron, so if you are on a low iron diet, do not exceed 4 teaspoons a day.

Matcha green tea

This is an absolute must. For all you coffee drinkers, this is a nice switch. We tend to drink coffee to get a pick-me-up. Matcha will give you the same effect, and is better for your health. You can get matcha green tea at Starbucks now. Matcha has a higher nutrient value than most other green teas. It's extremely high in antioxidants when these leaves are ground into a fine chlorophyll-rich powder. It does contain caffeine, but it is a different form of caffeine that will release energy over several hours. You will become more and more alert. I find that when I drink matcha, I just feel better. I have tried coffee a few times and always get the jitters. With matcha, you will get no jitters, and feel healthy. Caffeine drinks like coffee place stress on the adrenal glands. There is evidence that matcha will help with restoring hormonal balance, so it's actually beneficial to the adrenal glands.

Rooibos

Rooibos has been popular in Southern Africa for generations and is now consumed in many countries. Rooibos has anti-carcinogenic and anti-mutagenic effects. Rooibos tea is commonly used for its anti-inflammatory and anti-allergenic properties. It may offer relief from fever, asthma, insomnia, colic in infants, and skin disorders.

Rooibos is known for its high level of antioxidants and alkalizing properties. It does not contain caffeine like green tea. Try to use the whole ground leaves since most of the nutrients do not transfer to the water when the leaves are steeped. Rooibos extracts are also used in ointments for eczema.

White chai

White chai is a tea we are starting to hear more about in North America. It is grown in Peru in the Amazon and is extremely nutrient dense, packed with trace minerals, vitamins, and essential fats. It is great to add to your diet. White chai could be compared to flaxseed as both are high in omega-3. If you recall, flaxseed needs to be ground for optimum nutrition; white chai does not. White chai is loaded with antioxidants, has about 20 percent high-end proteins, and is packed with magnesium, potassium, calcium, and iron. White chai makes a very healthy choice, high in soluble and insoluble fiber. It will help keep up your energy and help you maintain a feeling of fullness. Sprinkle a tablespoon on your salads. It may be hard to find, but is becoming more common in your local health food stores.

Yerba mate

You may have heard of yerba mate. It is used in many weight loss products, and I am glad that certain brands have changed from unhealthy caffeine and other stimulants to yerba mate.

Yerba mate is very rich in chlorophyll, antioxidants, and trace minerals, and is great for digestion. Yerba mate does contain caffeine; however, it is one of the healthiest forms available. I call this "good caffeine". You can use yerba mate in many of your recipes. It will give you more stimulation and energy. I highly recommend this product to help you on your journey with weight loss.

Agave nectar

I love this natural sweetener as a replacement for honey and sugar. Throw all your other sweeteners away and change to this healthy alternative. Unfermented agave will give you a slow release of carbohydrates and trace minerals. This is a fantastic sweetener; use it for a healthier choice.

Apple cider vinegar

For those of you who just cannot give up your vinegar, change to apple cider vinegar. It is a little acidic, but once it enters the body it becomes alkaline-forming. This is great for salad dressings and sauces. Although it's made from fermented apples, it is by far a healthier vinegar choice. It's time to throw your white vinegar away.

Balsamic vinegar

Balsamic vinegar is easily accessible, and has an alkalizing effect on the body. Combine balsamic vinegar with hemp oil for a very healthy salad dressing.

Ginger

Ginger, to me, is a must-use. It has to be fresh ginger. It helps with digestion and upset stomach. Its anti-inflammatory properties help in the recovery of soft tissue injuries, and with long- term strain. You can put ginger in everything. I even put it in hot water and drink it.

Stevia

Stevia is another sweetener that I like. It is 25 times sweeter than sugar. When dried, it contains no carbohydrates, and therefore, will not have any effect on the body's insulin levels when ingested. It can even help stabilize other sugars and starch when consumed in the same sitting. Stevia has become mainstream and is the best choice instead of artificial sweeteners, as it is a whole food, ground into powder and dried. You can add it to many foods, including your protein shakes or smoothies, to help with sustained energy. Stevia is acidic in the body but better then regular sugar.

Important tips in your healthy eating program

Eating for life is not just about losing weight. Below, I have given you a series of recipes that are all alkalizing. It should not be difficult to introduce these into your diet. For example, an alkaline smoothie every day that tastes great is a very easy change to start with.

Eat often

We have all heard it over and over. You must eat often, five to six small meals per day, to lose weight. Why do we have to do this? When you go on a diet or cut your calories, your brain senses starvation, and sends a command through your body to store fat because famine is on its way. The key to getting fit is making sure your body does not go into starvation mode. There is only one way to do that and that is to eat frequently and often.

Healthy meals

If you fail to plan your meals, you're planning to fail. Before you start each day, plan exactly what you are going to eat. This is the best way to stop you from going out and eating junk food because you are hungry. Think about when you get really hungry. This is when you start to eat anything in sight. When you plan your meals, you tend not to overeat in one sitting. This is one of the major causes of weight gain and obesity around the world, eating over-sized portions.

How to eat less

This may seem weird, but it works if you trick your brain before you eat. If you have just a little bite of fat, you will want to eat less. But it should be the right kind of fat, not a doughnut. When you eat 12 almonds just 20 minutes before a meal, you trick your brain and slow your appetite. Now you can sit down to really enjoy a meal rather than eating just because you are starving.

How to become less hungry later in the afternoon

If you eat 30 grams of fiber per day, and consume most of it in the morning, it will make you less hungry late in the afternoon. It will slow down the transit of food across the ileocecal valve, keeping your stomach feeling fuller longer. A great way to start the day with enough fiber would be having whole grains, healthy cereal, or fruit.

The great thing about fiber is its helps lower blood sugar levels and decreases insulin levels. It has been shown to lower calorie intake for up to 18 hours a day. I suggest taking 1 to 2 grams of fiber before each meal and at bedtime, and gradually increase it up to 5 grams. Adding too much, too fast will result in gas.

Along with fiber, adding a red pepper to your daily eating plan early in the morning will help reduce your food intake later in the day. There is an ingredient in pepper called capsaicin, and many say that it will increase your metabolism and decrease your overall daily calorie intake.

Change your plates

We're accustomed to eating everything on our plate and truth is, everything has become bigger, including our plates. It is a major factor behind why society has grown so overweight. Many studies show we quite often don't feel satisfied until our plate is clean, no matter how big it is. Here is what you have to do: Go out and buy nine-inch plates. This does not mean you can load the food up so it hits your ceiling; your portion should be about the size of a fist.

Grapefruit aromatherapy oil

Yes, you heard me right. There have been numerous studies done on the scent of grapefruit oil, which helps reduce appetite and body weight. Perhaps while sniffing it, you can eat a grapefruit at the same time.

Who do you surround yourself with?

Studies show that if you have an overweight mate, there is a very good chance you will be overweight as well, and an even greater chance that you will have overweight children. The statement that "what you surround yourself with becomes your reality" is true in all areas of life. Broke people typically are not hanging out with millionaires. Quite often, people who are overweight have a lot of overweight friends as well.

A few powerful things to fight inflammation:

Inflammation is a major factor in weight loss. Omega-3 fatty acids are found in fish oils, and will help lower inflammation. You can get this in a few different ways. One is from eating good old fish. I would suggest you have three, four-ounce servings of fish per week. If you cannot do that, take 2 grams of fish oil capsules a day.

Green tea will also help with inflammation. Remember, the healthiest green tea is matcha. Studies have shown that if a person drinks three glasses of green tea per day, it will help you lose weight and shrink your waist circumference by 5 percent in three months. It will also speed up your metabolism.

The truth about TV

How many of you know that Oprah doesn't even watch TV? TV gives us the ability to sit around. Our hands do nothing, just waiting to pick up some kind of food. Most of us have been conditioned from a young age to watch TV and snack on junk food. We teach our kids how to do this because they watch us. The average child watches 17 hours of TV per week.

Cinnamon

Adding a half a teaspoon a day of cinnamon to your eating plan will help reduce those hunger cravings, and reduce blood pleasure and cholesterol levels. Cinnamon, for some strange reason, has a somewhat insulin-like effect.

Meditation

Studies show that meditation can greatly decrease your risk factor for coronary heart disease. The more you meditate, the greater chance you have of lowering blood pressure and insulin resistance.

Why do you gain weight when you miss meals?

As soon as you miss a meal, your body stops burning those calories off and starts storing them in not-so-attractive places. This is exactly why diets that deprive you don't work. When this happens, your body goes into famine mode, your metabolism slows right down, and your body stops burning calories. The key to weight loss is to burn off your calories before they can be turned into fat. You don't even have to be burning them off with exercise, you can burn them off by eating 5 to 6 small, healthy meals per day. Actually, your body burns most of your calories without you even knowing it, just from the energy you take to breathe, to sleep, and to think.

Are you an avoider?

There are many avoiders in the weight loss industry. What is an avoider? It is someone who gets off their healthy eating plan, and then gives up. We avoid what we have to do to live a healthy lifestyle. We don't want to be rejected, so we isolate ourselves from people. We stop talking about anything that has to do with health, and hope the challenges will just disappear. It is much easier to wolf down an ice cream cake than to face what we are avoiding.

Avoiders gain and lose, gain and lose, gain and lose. Avoiders don't just avoid their weight issues, they avoid having to deal with their expenses, taking care of their business, and even people who may want to help them. The bottom line is, avoiders work hard to separate themselves from any emotions that might be unpleasant.

The plan for a long, healthy life

At this point, you are probably wondering, what should I put on my plate? The key is to put electron-rich, green foods, and mono- and poly-unsaturated fats into your body. These are the foods that will maintain alkalinity in the body and build healthy blood. Have 70 percent of your plate covered with these foods; the rest of your plate can have grains, fish, beans, soy, and cooked vegetables. Have a big salad with every meal, with cooked or less alkaline foods on the side.

Most of us have been eating acidic food for years. Our taste buds have become accustomed to this way of eating. We start to crave this exact taste. If we had been conditioned to eat the other way, having a more alkaline diet, we then would crave more foods that are alkalizing rather than acidic. As you start to eat a more alkaline-based diet, you will lose the taste for acidic foods. The more acidic foods you eat, the more acidic foods you will crave. The more alkaline foods you eat, the more alkaline foods you will crave.

Once your body starts to become more alkaline, you will start to notice increased energy. And as your body becomes more energized, it will start to crave more energy and, therefore, crave foods that are more alkaline. You will notice as your overall health starts to operate at an optimum level that the acidic foods that have been bringing you down, making you tired and sick, will simply not appeal to you anymore.

In the end, because you are providing your body with

the nutrients that it really craves to live a long, healthy life, you require less food intake overall. You will do this unconsciously, and never feel unsatisfied. We all know that the less food we eat, the less weight we gain. As you follow this plan, you will watch the weight magically disappear. However, even more importantly, you will have a much better quality of life. This program is designed to keep disease out of your body, and help you live a long, healthy life.

The changing phase to better health

This plan is about helping your organs function the way they should. What you will do here is program yourself to start to become automatic in some of your choices so you can change patterns that have been holding you back. You must realize by now that weight problems stem from behaviors you choose over and over, year after year. When you program yourself to eat healthier foods each day, you will no longer feel the need to go out and binge on less healthy options. Let's face the facts. One of the major causes of overeating, or eating the wrong foods, is we don't have the time to prepare healthier options. However, eating healthier does not have to be time consuming. I have included recipes below that can be made in as few as 5 minutes. Others will take 15–30+ minutes. You can choose what you feel suits your needs the best.

So remember – you need to reprogram your brain to a new way of thinking. Getting in shape is not about counting calories and cutting carbs, it is about feeling full and satisfied. When you feel content, you are not going to go out and eat foods that are not good for you. This program is about eating foods that are nutritionally good for you, that will help to give you healthy cells; to keep disease out; to get you to start working on becoming full; and to stop eating when you shouldn't. It's important to start learning to listen to your brain when it gives you the signals that you are satisfied, and to not keep eating.

I am going to lay out a few different strategies to help you with your eating plan. This plan will teach you how to alkalize your body; remember, diseases can't live in an alkaline body. It is crucial for you to read over what some foods do in your body, and what alkaline and acidic really mean. For those people who just have to have meat, dairy, and other acid foods, the goal is to reduce these foods over time. You will notice that you will feel and look better, and have more energy.

It is s very important for you to understand that when you're finished the 90-day challenge, you will likely make mistakes, and start to get a little off track. I have designed the program so you can catch those old behaviors that may creep up and stop you from achieving success. It is important to recognize that when you start to get off track, it is possible to get back on track again. Catch yourself before you spin out of control and give up completely.

Step 1: Cleanse the body

Most people are shocked to learn that the average person holds between 5 and 10 pounds of putrefied fecal matter and other foul material in his or her body at one time. If you are determined to have optimum health, then the concept of doing a colon cleanse should appeal to you. If you would like more energy, I guarantee that when you get rid of that 5 to10 pounds lurking inside you, you will feel that much lighter.

A colon cleanse will start to eliminate toxins, dirt, waste, bacteria, and even parasites that have been stored in your digestive system. You will start to return to your natural state of balance, and feel refreshed. You will improve your skin quality, get rid of cellulite, reduce weight, enhance your immune system and, of course, increase your energy level. You don't have to do a colon cleanse to start this program, but I really think you should. It will help you lose weight faster.

Step 2: Not too many changes at one time

One of the surest ways to fail at a new program is to try to make too many changes at one time. That is why a lot of diets fail to give you long-term results. In this eating plan, we are teaching you how to eat to live a long, healthy life. The idea is not to eat just to lose weight, or eat because we need to eat, but to prevent many diseases by eating the right foods in the right quantities. When making the transition to a more alkaline way of eating, some may find more success by easing into it. For those who can make the full 360, go for it! Most of us, however, need to take a series of small steps that in the end will give your body big rewards. When you make small changes, there is a good chance you will stick with them long-term. We have to condition ourselves to a new way of doing things, and that takes some time. Moving toward an alkalizing lifestyle is a process. You will start to enjoy the journey because you will start to feel better and have more energy.

Now let me stress again that the foods you intake that are very acidic (such as meat and dairy) need to be reduced. I am not asking you to cut them out all at one time. I am asking you to start making more of your diet alkaline and less acidic. Eventually, you will start eating more alkaline foods more often because you will just start to feel better.

I care about you, and I care about the quality of life you are going to have as you get older. Although this is a weight loss program, it is just as much about getting your mind on the right track, and getting your body healthy inside so you can have the best quality of life possible.

The goal is to get to the point where you cover your plate with 70 percent alkaline foods and 30 percent acidic foods. To start with, cut back on things like meat and dairy. I am not saying you can't have these initially – just begin to cut back. I am teaching you how to start to create a healthy body from the inside out, and with a healthy body, you start to lose weight. Remember, the more alkaline your meals are, the easier it is to lose weight and the better you will feel. We're only as healthy as our cells, so the goal is to create healthy cells in your body. Gradually moving away from acidic foods will accomplish this.

Step 3: Eat the same meal every day

Studies show that people who eat the same meal every day will lose more weight than those who eat many different types of meals. This is a crucial step in this program because it helps you to unconsciously change behaviors and patterns.

The first 10 days you will eat the exact same breakfast, the next 10 days you will eat the exact same lunch, and for the following 10 days you will eat the exact same dinner. This meal has to be 70 percent alkaline and 30 percent acidic. Month two and month three will run the same way as month one. For the other meals, you will have a variety of choices.

Step 4: Why a healthy breakfast?

Breakfast is by far the most important meal of the day. The typical American diet consists of things like pancakes, syrups, white bread, butter, eggs, sausage, fruit juice, cold and hot cereals, bacon, coffee, and yogurt. It is probably the most highly acid of all the meals in our diet, yet this is the most important meal of your day.

It's hard to start your day at a highly effective level when your body contains yeast, fungus, and other microforms caused by eating these foods. When these huge quantities of sugar and carbohydrates enter the blood and tissues, they become acidic. Most of these breakfast foods have very little water content in them, and will also be highly constipating. Many have a dense source of protein, which will promote microform growth and will be high in parasite activity.

After you have a great night's sleep, your body needs to be taken care of in a much more delicate way to start your day. It amazes me how many people have to turn to coffee to start their day for that burst of energy, and who don't realize that a major crash is on its way. I have given you healthy teas that give you the same energy effect as coffee to start your day.

One of the easiest ways to change to a more alkalizing diet in the morning is to start integrating foods like buck-wheat. As a cereal grain, it will remind you of traditional cereal. At first, it may seem strange to eat things like a salad, vegetables, or a veggie wrap in the morning, but this is something you can get used to. You will feel so much better. If you are in a rush, a good, healthy, alkaline protein shake is a great way to start your day. I also suggest having a high fiber meal first thing in the morning. This will help you burn fat faster and stay fuller longer. So start your day with a higher fiber meal, but one that is lower in carbohydrates. You will notice that your blood sugar will not drop as fast throughout the day (as happens with a starchy, sugary breakfast). And you will have more energy to burn over a longer period of time. The majority of my clients who eat this way start to feel significantly better in the morning and have more energy. It's a lot easier to stick with something when it makes you feel great.

Step 5: Change the plate to 70/30

This is an extremely important part of the program, and extremely important to help you live a long, healthy life. Work to have each meal be at least 70 percent alkaline and 30 percent acidic on your plate. Most of our plates nowadays are 90 percent acidic and 20 percent alkaline. When you adjust this to 70/30, you don't have to cut calories or measure out things, just give the vegetables the spotlight on your plate.

We talked a lot about the importance of water and how your body needs it. Your body is 70 percent water. The earth is 70 percent water. Ensure your plate corresponds with 70 percent high water content foods that are alkalizing. When you change your plate to 70 percent alkaline and 30 percent acidic, you will notice the weight start to come off, but even better, you will start to feel better and add many healthy years to your life.

Below you will find charts ranking foods from the highest alkaline foods to the highest acidic foods. Work really hard to keep yourself in the more alkaline range. The eating plan I have given you is not hard to follow. If you sometimes don't have time to prepare meals, just look at the chart and grab some highly or moderately alkaline foods, for example, a handful of pumpkin seeds and a cucumber. Again the goal is to work to have your plate 70 percent high water alkaline foods. If you get into the habit of doing this, your energy will increase more than you have ever experienced. Your insides will feel fantastic and you will lose weight quickly, at the same time creating a healthy body and adding years to your life. Now that is a good eating plan to follow!

Highly alkaline foods

Dairy

- human breast milk

Vegetables

- cucumbers, kale, dandelion, green sea vegetables (such as agar, arame, dulse, hijiki, and nori), sprouted beans (including soy sprouts), parsley

Beans and legumes

- soy nuts, soy lecithin

Beverages

- alkaline water, fresh vegetable juice

Condiments

- sea salt, Celtic salt

Nuts and seeds

- pumpkin

Moderately alkaline foods

Vegetables

- tomato, avocado, green beans, sorrel, spinach, garlic, celery, cabbage, lettuce, bell peppers, collard greens, broccoli, endive, arugula, mustard greens, okra, radishes, salad greens, beets, onions

Beans and legumes

- edamane (green soy beans), lima beans, navy beans, white navy beans, granulated soy (cooked ground soy beans)

Condiments

- red pepper, cayenne, garlic, ginger, onion

Fruit

- avocados

Low alkaline foods

Dairy

- goat's milk

Vegetables

- Brussels sprouts, peas, asparagus, artichokes, comfrey, cauliflower, zucchini, rhubarb, leeks, watercress, chives, kohlrabi, carrots, sweet potatoes, rutabaga

Beans and legumes

- lentils, soy flour, tofu

Beverages

- distilled water

Condiments

- herbs and most spices

Nuts and seeds

- sesame, cumin, fennel, caraway, almonds (raw, unsalted)

Fruits

- cherries (sour) coconut, grapefruit, lemons, limes

Grains

- quinoa, buckwheat (groats or flour), spelt (grains or flour), spelt bread (yeast free, sugar free, and preservative free)

Low alkaline foods

Fats

- olive oil, borage oil, coconut oil, avocado oil, flaxseed oil, evening primrose oil, marine lipids, cod liver oil, almond oil, soy oil

Sweeteners

- stevia, chicory

Low acidic foods

Dairy

- soymilk, rice milk, milk, cream

Beans and legumes

- black beans, chick peas, seitan, kidney beans

Condiments

- curry powder

Nuts and seeds

- sunflower, flax, pecans, brazil nuts, hazelnuts

Fruits

- plums, fresh dates, nectarines, cantaloupe, sweet cherries

Grains

- millet, kasha, triticale, amaranth

Fats

- sunflower oil, grape seed oil, canola oil

Fish

- wild freshwater (not farm-raised)

Moderately acidic foods

Condiments

- ketchup, mayonnaise, vanilla, nutmeg, table salt

Nuts and seeds

- walnuts

Fruit

- oranges, bananas, pineapple, peaches, watermelon, honeydew, mango, apples, blackberries, fresh figs, dewberry, lingberry or longberry, guava, cherimoya, apricots, papayas, tangerines, currants, gooseberries, grapes, cranberries, strawberries, blueberries, raspberries, persimmons

- brown rice, wild rice, oats, rye bread, whole grain bread, whole-meal bread, wheat, biscuits

Fats

- margarine, butter, ghee, corn oil

Meat, poultry, fish

- wild ocean (not farm-raised)

Beverages

- fruit juice (natural, unprocessed)

Highly acidic foods

Dairy

- Cheese, cottage cheese, ice cream, yogurt, soy cheese, goat cheese, whey, casein (milk protein)

Vegetables

- mushrooms

Highly acidic foods

Beverages

- alcohol (including beer and wine), coffee, fruit juice (processed and sweetened), tea, soft drinks, sports drinks

Condiments

- mustard, vinegar, rice syrup, soy sauce, msg, jam, jelly, yeast, malt, cocoa, carob

Nuts and seeds

- pistachios, peanuts, cashews

Fruits

- All dried, pickled, or canned fruit

Grains

- barley (pearl or pot), oat bran, corn, rye

Sweeteners

- artificial sweeteners, saccharin, aspartame, white sugar, beet sugar, corn syrup, molasses

Meat, poultry and fish

- shellfish, farm-raised fish, pork, veal, beef, chicken, poultry, eggs, organ meats

The following are the most important to avoid – with better alternatives:

Avoid - Whole milk cheese
Better– light or nonfat cheese
A lot better - rice or soy cheese

Avoid - Whole eggs
Better - Egg whites
Even better – Egg beaters – made from real eggs

Avoid – whole milk
All right - skim milk
A lot better - soy milk, rice milk
Great - hemp milk or almond milk

Avoid - Ice cream
All right – nonfat frozen yogurt
A lot better - soy yogurt

Avoid - Beef or pork
All right – grain-fed chicken or turkey (white meat)
A lot better - soy-based meat alternatives

Avoid - Mayonnaise for salads
All right - Dijon mustard

Avoid – Whole mild yogurt
Not great – non-fat yogurt
A lot better - soy yogurt

I have talked a lot in this book about meat. By now you should have a better understanding of the consequences of eating too much meat. However, if you feel you must consume some meat, please limit the amount you consume. Definitely cut out red meats. Even though fish is acidic in the body, I still enjoy it – especially because it has so many other health benefits. If you have to eat meat, limit it to a maximum of a small portion once a day. If you can limit it throughout your week, even better.

Choose low-fat meats, such as skinless turkey and chicken. Choose leaner cuts of meat and avoid the well-marbled cuts. Avoid the meats that are surely hazardous to your long-term health, such as hot dogs, bacon, cold cuts, sausage, regular hamburgers, and spareribs. Make sure you trim all the fat off your meat before cooking it. This will prevent the fat from soaking in. Do not add bread crumbs to things like meatballs and meatloaf as they will soak up the fat in the food.

Work hard to switch to soy-based meat alternatives that are now in just about every grocery store. Remember, I used to eat meat three times per day, and lots of it. I made the change, and now I feel so much better. My increased energy level, never getting sick, and feeling like I am on top of the world could never compare to my state after I had put all that dead stuff in me. Once you try this, you will never go back.

The best meat, if you must eat meat:

If you are going to eat meat and poultry, eat organic, kosher meat. The typical animal has been tampered with in the breeding stage, and can never be natural. These animals are injected with growth hormones and antibiotics, which means the meat we eat is loaded with additives that can harm us. Animals are not allowed to roam freely or exercise normally, which in turn can create a buildup of toxins and disease. Imagine being caged and not allowed to roam freely your entire life. This could not be healthy for you. These animals are also fed an unnatural diet of chemicals and food that they would never eat naturally. Many cows are fed ground-up pig parts, goat parts, and horse parts. A lot of these animals used as feed are diseased and not fit for human consumption. Remember that the cow is a vegetarian and is not supposed to be eating diseased animals.

Typically, animals are slaughtered by being hit in the head. The animal experiences incredible pain and trauma. Adrenaline, which is highly poisonous, permeates the animal's tissue. The blood, which is also loaded with toxins, permeates the tissue. The animal will often die in its own urine and feces. Then the meat is typically aged, which means the flesh is hung in a dark room and allowed to rot. A green, toxic mold starts to cover the rotting flesh. This is nothing compared to the bacteria that covers the meat and fills it with more toxins.

The difference between this and organic or kosher meat

An organic animal has not been genetically modified and taken it out of its natural state. It has been given no drugs, so all the meat is drug-free. Organically-raised animals are allowed to graze the fields naturally. They grow at a normal rate, and are not filled with toxins or disease. The organic, grass-fed cow eats grass from nature as it should. The grass has not been filled with chemicals, fertilizers, herbicides, or pesticides.

An organic animal that is kosher is killed in the most humane way possible, usually by slicing its throat. There is no pain, and the blood is immediately drained out. Its internal organs are inspected to make sure it is 100 % healthy, and the tissue is salted to draw out any blood and kill any bacteria. It is not aged.

Remember, I am not asking you to give up everything. I am just showing you some healthier options. Organic, kosher meat is still acidic, so make sure you completely alkalize yourself. Start to limit the servings you have. It is your choice what kind of life you want to live.

On a budget

If you are on a budget, it is actually cheaper to eat more alkaline food. Some of the recipes are very cheap, and others cost only a little more than what you are spending now. However, if you shop around for alkaline foods, you can save some money. A handful of carrots, a few dates, and a glass of lemon water do not cost that much.

Thirty minutes before each meal, have a big glass of water with lemon in it. Lemon water is highly alkaline, and this will help you eat less and fill you up faster.

Example of a 10-day Eating Plan:

Day 1

Breakfast: Smoothie (p.228)

Snack: Energy bar (p.227)

Lunch: Fast wraps (p.218)

Snack: Fast nut snack (Almonds, unsalted or soy nuts) (full or half grapefruit optional)

Dinner: Hearty squash quesadillas (p.218)

Day 2

Breakfast: Smoothie (p.228)

Snack: Cantaloupe and veggies

Lunch: Sprouted bread or whole-grain bagel with salmon, veggies on the side with your choice of healthy dressings.

Snack: Energy bar (p.227)

Dinner: Fabulous fajitas (p.217)

Day 3

Breakfast: Smoothie (p.228)

Snack: Fast nut snack with vegetables (optional)

Lunch: Veggie burger on sprouted bread (not fully alkaline) with salad or vegetables

Snack: Energy bar (p.227)

Dinner: Healthy quinoa pizza (p.217)

Day 4

Breakfast: Smoothie (p.228)

Snack: Energy bar (p.227)

Lunch: Healthy avocado burritos (p.219)

Snack: Grapefruit and veggies

Dinner: Quinoa wrap (p.212)

Day 5

Breakfast: Smoothie (p.228)

Snack: Fast nut snack

Lunch: Alkaline sandwich, cantaloupe

Snack: Strawberry blueberry pudding (p.224)

Dinner: Salmon, wild rice, vegetable (preferably raw)

Day 6

Breakfast: Smoothie (p.228)

Snack: Cantaloupe and veggies

Lunch: Alfalfa sprouts salad (p.212)

Snack: Almond butter on celery

Dinner: Healthiest burgers not alive (p.215)

Other options: veggie burgers, highly acidic lean meat burger (preferably organic) —— just remember to work to keep your plate 70 percent alkaline.

Day 7

Breakfast: Smoothie (p.228)

Snack: Grapefruit and veggies

Lunch: Alkaline sandwich, piece of cantaloupe

Snack: Energy bar (p.227)

Dinner: Split pea soup (p.222)

Day 8

Breakfast: Smoothie (p.228)

Snack: Energy bar (p.227)

Lunch: Sprouted wheat salad (p.211)

Snack: Handful of dates and veggies

Dinner: Happy jambalaya (p.216)

Day 9

Breakfast: Smoothie (p.228)

Snack: Grapefruit and veggies

Lunch: Cayenne avocado salad with balsamic dressing (p.211)

Snack: Energy bar (p.227)

Dinner: Chow mein tofu (p.216)

Day 10

Breakfast: Smoothie (p.228)

Snack: Handful of dates

Lunch: Sprouted wheat salad (p.211)

Snack: Cantaloupe and veggies

Dinner: Fish fillet, (not fully alkaline), broccoli, brown rice

RECIPES

Breakfast

Buckwheat pancakes with raw almond butter and fruit or almond butter from the store (not as alkaline as home-made, but still good.)

You will find that these pancakes are much more healthy and filling than any others made with refined carbohydrates. You want to cook these at a low temperature so the fatty acids in the pancakes are not destroyed at a high heat, taking away the good nutrients. A healthier choice to maple syrup is to use agave nectar as an alternative.

Cooking instructions: In a food processor, process all ingredients until smooth. Lightly oil a pan with coconut oil and heat over medium heat. Pour batter in and cook until bubbles arise, or cook for 5 minutes. Turn over and cook for another 5 minutes.

These pancakes are a lot healthier than traditional pancakes and come very close to the same taste. Sprinkle with cinnamon and nutmeg to really get the traditional taste of pancakes.

Buckwheat Pancakes

1 cup buckwheat flour, ¼ cup ground flaxseed, ¼ cup hemp flour, 2 tsp baking powder, 1 tsp cinnamon, ½ tsp nutmeg, 1 banana, 2 cups of water, ½ cup barley flakes (or buckwheat, sprouted or cooked)

Mix buckwheat flour, flaxseed, hemp flour, baking powder, cinnamon and nutmeg in a bowl. In the processor, process the banana and water and add all dry ingredients, until mixture is smooth. Stir in barley flakes with a spoon.

Makes 2 large servings

Blueberry Pancakes

You will find these blueberry pancakes very similar to the blueberry pancakes that you are accustomed to, with one exception: they have 100 percent better nutrient value.

2 fresh or soaked dried dates, 1 cup blueberries, 1 cup of hemp milk, ¾ cup of water, ½ cup of buckwheat flour, ½ cup sprouted or cooked quinoa, 1 tsp baking powder, 1 tsp baking soda, sea salt to taste

Makes 2 large servings

Chocolate Banana Pancakes

If you don't make these for yourself, at least make them for your kids. Your kids will love them, and they're extremely healthy, filled with vitamins, minerals, essential fatty acids, and high quality protein.

2 bananas, 2 fresh or soaked dried dates, 1 cup popped amaranth, (amaranth is a great substitute for flour in pancakes),1 cup chocolate hemp milk, 1 cup of water, ½ cup buckwheat flour, ¼ cup ground flaxseed, ¼ cup hemp flour, ¼ cup roasted carob powder, ¼ cup unsweetened carob chips, sea salt to taste

Makes 2 large servings

Pear Ginger Banana Cereal

This is a great substitute for many grocery store cereals that are laced with sugars and refined grains.

1 banana, 1 pear, 1 date, ¼ cup almonds, 1 tbsp ground flaxseed, 1 tbsp hemp flour, ½ tbsp roasted carob powder, ½ tbsp grated fresh ginger

Makes 1 large serving

Toasted Cinnamon Apple Cereal

I love this recipe for breakfast since it's loaded with fiber, and breakfast is the most important meal in which to have lots of fiber. You can also make a big batch of this and put it in your fridge for up to 2 weeks. This is a very easy breakfast to eat for 10 days in a row.

½ apple diced, 1 cup oats (gluten-free, add sprouted or cooked quinoa), ½ cup diced almonds, ½ cup ground flaxseed, ½ cup hemp flour, ½ cup unhulled sesame seeds, ½ cup sunflower seeds, ½ tsp cinnamon ¼ tsp nutmeg, ¼ tsp ground stevia leaf, ¼ tsp sea salt, ¼ cup hemp oil, ¼ cup molasses, 2 tbsp apple juice

Preheat oven to 250° F

Blend together hemp oil, molasses, and apple juice. Combine apple, oats, almonds, ground flaxseed, hemp flour, sesame seeds, sunflower seeds, cinnamon, nutmeg, stevia, and sea salt. Mix well all liquid and dry ingredients.

Use coconut oil to spread on a baking tray (lightly oiled). Bake for 1 hour and let cool.

Makes about 5 servings.

Eggless option

I don't eat eggs, as they are very acid-forming in the body. This dish is loaded with fiber from vegetables. The tofu gives you lean protein and calcium.

8oz firm tofu, crumbled, 1sp ground turmeric, 1 tsp celtic sea salt, ½ tsp ground cumin (optional), 4 tomatoes, quartered, 2 tbsp extra virgin olive oil, 1 large onion, chopped, 1 small sweet potato, chopped (optional), 2 stalks of celery, chopped, 1 red bell pepper, chopped

I included turmeric, as it is a spice that is well used in Indian food and is a natural anti-inflammatory.

Combine tofu, turmeric, salt, and cumin in a bowl.

Puree tomatoes in a blender or food processor.

Heat oil over low to medium heat in a large skillet. Sauté onions until softened. Add sweet potato, if using, sauté until tender. Add seasoned tofu and sauté until you have heated it through. Stir in tomato puree, cover and cook for 5 to 10 minutes or until tomato puree is heated thoroughly and flavors are blended.

Serves 4

Steel Cut Oats

Bob's Red Mill organic steel cut oats. Follow directions on package. Slightly acidic, but go for it.

Almond milk or rice milk

Raisins and cinnamon

Avocado Blueberry Extreme

This is a quick and easy breakfast to prepare and can also be eaten as a dessert.

1 avocado, peeled and pitted
Juice of ½ lemon
1 cup of frozen blueberries

Apple and Quinoa

½ cup of quinoa
1 apple
½ lemon
Cinnamon

Optional: raisins

Serves 2

Cook the quinoa according to instructions.

Grate the apple, cook it for a further 30 seconds, grate in the zest of the lemon and squeeze a little lemon in to taste. Add a sprinkle of cinnamon. Can add raisins.

Hearty Buckwheat Cereal

4 servings

1 cup buckwheat groats
2 1/2 cups water
1/2 teaspoon sea salt

Bring all ingredients to a boil, then cover and simmer for 30 minutes, stirring occasionally. Top with fresh fruit and almond milk.

Quick toast

Go with essence, manna or sprouted grain breads. (See breads)

Toast with almond butter. (vegetables on the side)

Breads

If you are going to choose bread, the best will be sprouted grain. The fewer the ingredients, the more natural they will be. Breads that use sprouted grain do not use flour so it's a healthier option. The bakery takes the grain and instead of grinding it up into flour, it sprouts the grain and then grinds that up. Because of the sprouting, these breads are more nutritious and they're cooked on low temperatures. You can find them in the frozen section of your health store. And not just breads, you can also find sprouted bagels and tortilla wraps.

Essence or manna bread comes close to being the most perfect bread on the planet. Essence bread is produced with sprouted grain berries and pure water. Most of our bread today is prepared with bleached and demineralized white flour, often polluted water, hydrogenated vegetable oil, yeast or baking soda, lard or butter, and chemical-laden table salt – all not good for our health. Healthier whole grain breads have now been introduced to the market, but there is just nothing that can compare to essence or manna bread. Essence or manna bread can be bought in most health food stores (in the freezer) or on the Internet. They're usually more expensive because they take more care and time to produce. You can also get sprouted wraps and tortillas. Costco now carries a sprouted grain bread.

Next best would be whole grain bread. Make sure its 100% whole grain. Read the labels before buying to make sure. Whole grain wraps, whole grain tortillas, whole grain bagels. These are moderately acidic but a lot better choice than white breads and whole wheat options. Stick to the 100 percent whole grains.

You can't go wrong with spelt breads and I enjoy the taste a lot more.

Salads

Sprouted Wheat Salad
Serves 6

3 cups fresh wheat sprouts (or any type of sprouts)
1 cup grated carrots
3/4 cup minced onion
3 tbsp flaxseed oil
1 1/2 tbsp fresh lemon juice

Mix all. Sprinkle with paprika. Serve on heavy greens.

Cayenne Avocado Salad
½ avocado, sliced; 1 sheet nori, chopped; 4 cups mixed greens; 1 tbsp nutritional yeast; ½ tsp. cayenne pepper.

Mix all. Sprinkle with paprika. Serve on bed of lettuce.

Alfalfa Sprout Salad
Serves 6

3 cups alfalfa sprouts
3 cups summer squash, chopped
2 red peppers, diced
2 green onions, chopped
1/4 cup onion, chopped

Dressing
Flaxseed oil, fresh lemon juice

Quinoa wrap

2 tomatoes, 1 avocado, 1 cucumber, 1 large carrot, 2 strips of dulse (tightly packed, ¼ cup) 1 cup soaked or cooked quinoa, 1 leaf of dinosaur kale, balsamic salad dressing

Peel avocado and cube, slice cucumber and tomatoes, grate carrots. Place all ingredients on the leaf of kale.

Bean Spinach Salad

1 (15 ounce) can pinto beans, rinsed & drained
1 (15 ounce) can chick peas, rinsed & drained
1 (15 ounce) can cannellini beans, rinsed & drained
1 red bell pepper, chopped
2 carrots, peeled & chopped
2 stalks celery, chopped
2 green onions, chopped (optional)
1/2 cup olive oil
2 tbsp flaxseed oil-optional
1 tbsp hemp oil-optional
2 tbsp fresh lime juice
2 tbsp lemon juice
2 tbsp agave syrup
1/2 tbsp celtic salt or sea salt
1-2 cloves minced garlic
1/4 cup chopped fresh cilantro
1/2 tbsp ground cumin

1 tsp ground black pepper
1 tsp chili powder
Cayenne pepper to season at serving time

1. In a large bowl, combine beans, chopped veggies, chives
2. In a large measuring cup, whisk together remaining ingredients
3. Pour dressing over vegetables and combine without mashing the beans
4. Serve over fresh greens

Serves 6-8

Quick Tuna Salad

1 can of chickpeas (drained)
1/2 cup of Veganaise mayo (moderately acidic)
1/2 red bell pepper, chopped
1 carrot, chopped
1 celery stalk, chopped
1/4 cup red onion, chopped
1 tbsp dried parsley

Juice from 1/2-1 lemon
Sea salt and black pepper to taste

You will not believe there is no tuna.

Healthy Guacamole Salad

Serves 2 to 4

3 avocados, finely chopped; 4 tomatoes, diced; ½ tablespoon garlic, minced; 1 bunch cilantro, chopped; ¼ to ½ pound baby romaine, mesclun, or regular romaine lettuce, chopped; juice of 1 lime; 2 tablespoons agave nectar or 1 stevia pack; celtic sea salt and freshly ground pepper to taste

Mix and enjoy

Beet Salad

2 to 4 servings

1 large beet, thinly sliced; 6 to 8 thin slices cantaloupe or 4 figs, quartered; squeeze of lemon juice, drizzle of olive oil, celtic sea salt and freshly ground pepper to taste, drizzle of agave nectar

Place slices of beets on plate; add lemon, oil, salt, pepper and agave.

Entrées

Mac and cheese

Not alkalizing, but a far better choice than the traditional macaroni and cheese. Great alternative to feed your kids.

12-16 oz cooked whole grain or spelt macaroni
1qt (4cups) rice milk or almond milk
4tbsp Earth Balance (soy free)
1/3 cup spelt flour
3 cups Daiya shredded cheddar or soy
1 cup Daiya shredded Italian blend
½ tsp pepper
1 tsp sea salt

Cook macaroni 6-8minutes. Heat the milk in a small saucepan, do not boil. Melt the Earth Balance in the same pot as macaroni was cooked in. Add the spelt flour and cook over low heat for 2 minutes, stirring constantly. Add hot milk, cooking for 2 more minutes. Take pan off the heat. Add the cheddar and Italian blend cheese, pepper and salt. Add the cooked macaroni and stir very well.
Pour into a baking dish. Bake for 30 minutes at 375 degrees.

Daiya brand products do not contain many of the common allergens, such as soy, dairy (casein or lactose), gluten, egg, peanuts, or tree nuts (excluding coconut).

Healthiest Burgers Not Alive

These are the healthiest and fastest burgers to make. They take about 10 minutes to make and when you do not cook them you leave their enzyme content intact. However, they are still very nutritious when cooked. I eat them raw about 70 percent of the time. These are very nutrient dense patties and will be quite filling with just a salad. You can use a whole grain or sprouted bun.

Makes 2 medium patties

Flaxseed Almond Burger

2 cloves garlic, 1 cup almonds, ½ cup ground flaxseed, 2 tbsp balsamic vinegar, 2 tbsp coconut oil or hemp oil, sea salt for taste

Makes 2 medium patties

Hemp Walnut Burger

1 cup of walnuts, ½ cup hemp seeds, 2 tbsp apple cider vinegar, 2 tbsp coconut oil or hemp oil, ½ tsp basil, ½ tsp oregano, sea salt for taste

Fish Fillet
Serves 2

1 48ml. box of coconut cream, ¾ tsp. real salt, ¼ tsp. pepper or cayenne or zip, ½ lemon juiced

For 2 hours, marinate fish in the refrigerator. Cook fish on low-medium heat in saucepan, flip over for 1 to 3 minutes and let the fish absorb the flavor of the sauce.

Chow Mein Tofu
Serves 4-6

2 boxes of tofu; 3 onions, cut into strips; 4 garlic cloves, minced; 1 tsp. gingerroot, grated; 6 celery stalks, thinly sliced; 2 carrots, thinly sliced; 1 cup pure water; 1tsp real salt; 1 can bean sprouts or 1 1/2 cups fresh; 1 can water chestnuts, sliced; 1 can bamboo shoots, 2 tsp. arrowroot powder, 1/4 cup pure water

Preheat oven to 400° F, and cut tofu into 1 ½ inch cubes. Spread cubes on oiled baking pan; bake for 30 minutes until brown. Sauté onions, garlic, and ginger. Add celery, carrots, water, and salt, and steam fry for 2 minutes. Add, just to warm, bean sprouts, bamboo shoots, and water chestnuts. Mix together arrowroot powder and 1/4 cup water. Add to vegetables to thicken broth. Add tofu. Serve over wild or brown rice, or quinoa.

Happy Jambalaya
Serves 6

1 cup long grain rice
14 ounces cooked kidney beans (rinse well, if canned)
1 yellow onion, finely diced
1 red bell pepper, finely chopped
1 green bell pepper, finely chopped
1 carrot, finely chopped
1 rib of celery, finely chopped
Kernels from 1 corn cob (about 1 cup)
2 cloves of garlic
1/4 to 1/2 tsp of cayenne pepper
1 tsp dried oregano
1/2 tsp ground black pepper
2 to 2 1/4 cups vegetable broth
Extra virgin olive oil
Handful of fresh parsley or cilantro, roughly chopped
Sea salt

1. Drizzle enough olive oil into a large pan to lightly cover the bottom, and set heat to between low and medium.

2. Add rice and sauté for about 5 minutes, then add onion and cook for another 2 minutes. Be sure to stir from time to time.

3. Add the rest of the vegetables, plus garlic, black pepper, oregano, and cayenne, and cook for another 2 minutes, stirring regularly.

4. Now the relaxing part: add between 1.5 to 2 cups of broth. Cover with a lid and bring to a boil. As soon as it reaches a boil, lower heat and allow to simmer for about 35 to 40 minutes. You don't want the ingredients to get dry and burn, so check on it at the 15–20-minute mark, and add a little extra broth if you don't see any liquid.

5. Once it's finished cooking, add kidney beans and give everything a good toss to allow the kidney beans to heat through. Season with sea salt, to taste.

Healthy Quinoa Pizza

Crust
1 cup cooked or sprouted adzuki beans, 1 cup cooked or sprouted quinoa, ½ cup ground sesame seeds, ¼ cup coconut oil or hemp oil, 2 tbsp dulse flakes

Using a food processor, process all ingredients until mixture balls up. Oil the tray with coconut oil (lightly). Spread mixture across tray. Choose thickness you prefer. Spread sundried spicy tomato sauce on crust (see spices), add toppings. Bake for 45 minutes. Watch when baking. Baking time will vary depending on the vegetables and how crisp you prefer the crust.

Fabulous fajitas (serves 2-4)

1tsp dried basil, ½ tsp ground cumin, ½ tsp chili powder, ¼ tsp vegetable salt, 8 oz tofu, cut into ½ inch strips, 2 tbsp extra virgin olive oil, 1 small onion, diced, 1 red pepper, diced, 1 large tomato, diced, 4 sprouted grain or brown rice tortillas

Fast Wraps

1 to 2 carrots, shredded, ½ cucumber, sliced, ½ red or green bell pepper, sliced into strips, 1 to 2 tomatoes, sliced, 2 to 4 sprouted grain or brown rice tortillas

In the middle of each tortilla spread the guacamole, place vegetables in the middle of the wrap and roll.

Hearty Squash Quesadillas

1 large onion, chopped, 2 red bell peppers, diced, 1 tbsp extra virgin olive oil, 1 pack of sprouted grain or brown rice tortillas

Using a large skillet, heat oil over medium heat for 5 minutes, sauté onion for 10 to 15 minutes, sauté red peppers until they have softened and onions have browned. Place tortilla on each plate. Spread sauce over each tortilla. Put red pepper mix and onion over half tortilla. For taste, add salt. Place tortilla in skillet folded in half. Cook till warm, turning one time.

Special sauce

Serving size, 2 cups

1 small butternut squash, peeled and cubed; add celtic sea salt. In saucepan, place squash, cover with water, and bring to a boil. Reduce heat to low, let simmer for about 10 to 15 minutes or until tender. Once done, drain.

Blend with food processor, blender, or hand-held blender until smooth. Season with salt.

Healthy Avocado Burritos

1/2 large or 1 small ripe avocado (a ripe avocado should yield under the pressure of your thumb)
1/2 tsp. organic onion powder
1/4 tsp. Celtic sea salt
1 tsp. lemon juice
2 or more fresh romaine lettuce leaves
1/4 cup of your favorite raw organic salsa from the health food store, or fresh, chopped tomatoes

Use a fork to mash the avocado and seasonings. Place the guacamole in the lettuce leaf and top with salsa or tomatoes and sprouts. Wrap it up and eat it like a burrito. **Stretch those avocados! If you just don't have enough ripe avocados to make guacamole, here's a little trick: For every medium avocado you use, blend 1 stalk of celery and 2 tsp. avocado or olive oil until creamy. Then mix with the avocado (a great way to get kids to eat celery, too).

Green Stir Fry with Mushroom & Red Onion

For main or side dish
1 serving

1 bunch of Swiss chard or other greens (collard, mustard, etc.)
1 cup sliced mushrooms
1 medium red onion, sliced
2 tbsp oil (your choice)
Braggs Amino Acids to taste
2 cloves garlic, sliced, chopped, or crushed
Salt and pepper to taste

Heat oil in a frying pan. Add garlic and onions, sauté. Add mushrooms and chopped greens. Cook for about 5 minutes. Add Braggs, salt and pepper, and serve.

Spicy Eggplant Pasta
Serves 2

7 oz. (200g) spelt pasta, 1 fresh eggplant, 1 fresh red bell pepper, 1 medium onion, 1 clove of garlic, 1 small chili, 1 cup yeast-free vegetable stock, 1 handful of fresh basil, ½ teaspoon organic sea salt, 1 pinch of cayenne pepper, extra virgin olive oil

Cut peppers and eggplant into cubes; chop onion, garlic, chili, and basil into small pieces. Heat olive oil in pan. Stir fry garlic and onions for a few minutes. Add pepper cubes, eggplant, and chili, and stir fry for another 2 to 3 minutes. Dissolve yeast-free vegetable stock in cup of water (see directions) and add to pan. Simmer on low for approximately 10 minutes. Occasionally stir. Add basil and season with cayenne pepper and salt. Pour sauce over pasta.

Sweet Potatoes

6 large sweet potatoes
1 ½ to 2 cups fresh coconut milk
1 tbsp extra virgin olive oil
1 tbsp sea salt
1 pinch of pepper
½ tbsp curry powder

Wash and chop the sweet potatoes and boil them for around 20 minutes.

Then mash the sweet potatoes to desired consistency and add the remaining ingredients.

Original Sweet Potatoes

1 ½ cups sweet potatoes, peeled and chopped
1 ½ cups cauliflower chopped
1 cup pine nuts
¼ cup leeks, chopped
2 tbsp onion powder
3 tbsp flaxseed oil
¼ cup filtered water
½ tbsp Celtic salt
2 tbsp dried parsley

In food processor, combine all ingredients and blend. Continue by pouring mixture into a high-speed blender, and blend until completely smooth. Adjust salt to taste.

Whole Grain Lasagna

6 servings

12 spelt or whole grain lasagna noodle strips, cooked al dente; pasta sauce (see pasta sauce); 4 to 6 ounces raw goat cheese, grated; 1 clove garlic, chopped; 1 zucchini, thinly sliced lengthwise; 1 eggplant, sliced lengthwise; 10 fresh spinach leaves; ¾ cup packed fresh basil; freshly ground black pepper to taste

Preheat oven to 350° F. In large baking dish, layer lasagna strips, tomato sauce, goat cheese, garlic, vegetables, basil and pepper. Bake for 25 minutes. Top with fresh basil.

Simple pizza

Makes 6

1 sprouted grain tortilla, 3 tbsp pasta sauce, 10 fresh basil leaves, 2 ounces raw cheddar style goat cheese.

Put tortilla in skillet. Spoon pasta sauce evenly on tortilla. Spread basil on top of sauce, sprinkle cheese on top of basil leaves. Place pan over heat until cheese melts. Remove and serve.

Soups

Pea soup

Serves 4
2 carrots, peeled
2 celery stalks, cut as desired
6 sprigs parsley
1 onion, chopped
4 cups water
2 cups crisp-steamed green beans
1 1/2 cups crisp-steamed asparagus
Dash of mace
1 bay leaf
1 tsp. vegetized or real salt

In food processor, chop all vegetables and add to 4 cups of water or vegetable stock in a soup pot. Cook until vegetables are softened – about 8-10 minutes – then place contents into a blender and puree until thick, creamy texture is achieved. Add sea salt and seasonings. Serve warm.

Sweet Potato and Carrot Bisque

Serves 4

2 sweet potatoes, 2 cups baby carrots, 1 cup of water, 2 cups vegetable broth, ½ tsp celtic sea salt, 1 packet stevia, ¼ tsp cumin, ½ tsp ground coriander, ¼ tsp minced ginger, ¼ tsp minced garlic

I love this recipe because there is no chopping of vegetables. Boil carrots and bake the sweet potatoes until soft. Mix all ingredients in a blender and process until uniform. Pour mixture in large saucepan, and heat.

Cantaloupe Soup

Serves 4

1 cantaloupe, ½ tsp cinnamon, ½ tsp nutmeg, ½ tsp garam masala, ½ tsp curry powder.

In a blender, combine all ingredients until smooth. Serve chilled in a bowl.

Thai Carrot Soup

15 carrots, cut into 1- to 2-inch slices; 32 ounces vegetable broth; 2 tbsp lemon grass; 1 small Spanish onion, chopped; 3 tbsp curry (or to taste); 3 tbsp minced ginger; 2 to 3 cloves garlic; fresh cilantro

Into a soup pot, place onion, lemon grass, broth, and carrots. Bring to a boil, and let simmer until carrots are soft. Put into blender and puree. When pureed, add curry. Add ginger and garlic to taste.

Raw Green Soup

1-2 avocados
1-2 cucumbers, peeled and seeded
1 jalapeno pepper, seeded
1/2 yellow onion, diced
Juice of 1/2 lemon
1-2 cups light vegetable stock or water
3 cloves roasted garlic
1 tbsp fresh cilantro
1 tbsp. fresh parsley
1 carrot, finely diced

Puree all ingredients (except onions and carrots) in a food processor. Add water for the consistency you like. Add carrots and onions.

Desserts

Strawberry blueberry pudding

1 avocado, peeled and pitted, 1 8oz container (about 10 medium) fresh strawberries, hulled, ½ cup frozen blueberries, 30 drops liquid stevia

Dessert on the Road

Serves 1 to 2

Juice of ¼ lemon, drizzle of agave nectar, 2 bananas sliced

On top of the banana, squeeze lemon juice and agave nectar. Great with a few dates.

Raw Chocolate Cake

Serves 10

1/2 cup cocoa powder
1/2 cup carob
1/2 cup finely ground almonds
1/3 cup agave syrup
1/4 cup coconut or cacao butter
Pinch of sea salt
For the chocolate filling
2 cups cocoa powder
1.5 cups agave syrup
1 cup coconut or cacao butter
1 tbsp vanilla extract (optional)
1 tbsp Lucama powder (optional)
1 tsp maca powder (optional)
For garnishing: strawberries, raspberries, or oranges

Crust

Combine all ingredients by hand or using a standing mixer. It will end up having a dough-like consistency. Spread the dough evenly into a 7-inch tart pan (a removable bottom or flexible silicon pans are simplest). Place in fridge for at least an hour.

Filling

Blend ingredients in a blender until smooth. Poor into the cake crust. Place cake back in the fridge and chill for about an hour.

Raw Chocolate Pudding

Makes 2 cups

Meat of 2 coconuts (or ½ an avocado), 6 dates, 4 tablespoons pure cocoa powder

Blend all ingredients in a food processor until smooth

Chocolate Shake

Serves 4

¼ cup pure cocoa powder, ½ cup almond milk, 1 young coconut or 1/8 avocado, 1 tsp vanilla extract, 2 trays of ice, 8 packets of stevia.

Blend until all ingredients are smooth.

Date and Pecan Pie Crust

Makes 1 crust

6 dates pitted, ½ cup pecans or walnuts, ¼ cup of almond milk, ½ tsp vanilla extract, ¼ tsp nutmeg, ¼ tsp of cinnamon, ¼ tsp ground cloves

In food processor, blend dates, nuts, almond milk, vanilla extract, and spices until uniform. Place in pie pan and press firmly. Fill the raw pie filling with fruit of your choice.

Ice cream (raw but not fully alkaline; 100 % better choice than traditional ice cream)

Makes about 4 cups

Chocolate Ice Cream

3 bananas, 3 tbsp pure cocoa powder, 2 tbsp organic, raw, unsalted tahini, 8 packets of stevia, 6 organic dates pitted, 3-4 cups ice cubes (about 14 cubes)

In blender, place bananas, cocoa powder, tahini, stevia, dates, and ¼ of the ice in a blender. Slowly add remaining ice cubes as it keeps blending. You want to use all the ice but may have to run it 2 or 3 times to use up all ice. You might want to use a small amount of coconut water to facilitate blending.

Strawberry Ice Cream

Makes about 4 cups

Meat of 2 young coconuts, 2 bags frozen organic strawberries, 8 packets stevia, 6 dates, pitted, 1 tsp organic
strawberry extract, 4 cups ice cubes (about 14 cubes)

In a blender, place coconut meat, strawberries, stevia,
dates, strawberry extract, and 1 cup of ice. Blend very
well. You may have to use all the ice to make it thick
enough, but it's not necessary. You might want to use a
small amount of coconut water to facilitate blending.

Energy Bars

If you're in a rush, you can pick up healthy, raw hemp
energy bars at your local health food store and some
supermarkets.

Pear Energy Bar

1 small pear, cored; ¾ fresh or soaked dried dates; ½
cup sunflower seeds; ¼ cup ground flaxseed; ¼ cup
hemp flour; ¼ cup walnuts; 2 tbsp grated fresh ginger;
sea salt; 2 tsp sesame seeds

Process all ingredients together in food processor, except
the sesame seeds. Before shaping into bars cover mixture in sesame seeds.

Makes approximately 12 1 3/4 ounce bars

Cinnamon Apple Energy Bar

1 small apple, cored, 1 cup fresh or soaked dried dates,
½ cup soaked or cooked quinoa, ¼ cup almonds, ¼ cup
ground flaxseed, ¼ cup hemp flour, 2 tsp cinnamon, ½
tsp nutmeg, sea salt

Makes approximately 12 1 3/4 ounce bars

Coconut Energy Bar

¾ cups fresh or soaked dates, ½ cup chopped mango, ½ cup ground flaxseed, ½ cup soaked or cooked quinoa, ¼ cup macadamia nuts, 1 tsp cinnamon, 1 tsp lemon zest, sea salt to taste, ¼ cup shredded coconut

Process all ingredients together except for coconut. Take mixture out from food processor, and work coconut into it by hand.

Makes approximately 12 1 3/4 ounce bars

Smoothies

Directions

Blend all ingredients together in a blender

All smoothies can stay in the fridge for about 3 days but are better when fresh. Here is a good tip to add to your smoothies when you feel really hungry. Add sprouted buckwheat or other pseudo-grains. Most smoothies have hemp protein in them. For a super fast drink, add a few scoops of hemp protein into the blender and add fresh or frozen fruit. Look for frozen fruit that does not contain any preservatives. Add any vegetables you would like as well. Get into the habit of having at least one smoothie per day. This will help you live longer and lose weight. When I am really busy, I may even have two or three in a day. It's better to get a quick, healthy smoothie than to miss a meal. This will stop you from going to the drive-thru and getting junk food. When I am busy, I pack two smoothies with me to last the day and a couple of healthy energy bars. This stops me from choosing bad foods when I get hungry. Each Smoothie recipe yields about two servings if prepared as directed.

Pear and Ginger Smoothie
1 banana; ½ pear, cored; 2 cups cold water (1 ½ cups water, plus 1 cup ice); 1 tbsp ground flaxseed;1 tbsp hemp protein; 1 tbsp. grated ginger

---

Chocolate Smoothie
1 banana, 2 fresh or soaked dates, 2 cups of cold water (or add 1 cup of ice and 1 ½ cups of water), ¼ cup almonds (or 2 tbsp raw almond butter), 1 tbsp ground flaxseed, 1 tbsp hemp protein, 1 tbsp roasted carob powder (healthy alternative to chocolate)

Pineapple Smoothie
1 banana, 2 fresh or soaked dates, 2 cups cold water (or add 1 cup of ice and 1 ½ cups of water), ½ medium papaya, ½ cup pineapple, 1tbsp ground flaxseed, 1 tbsp hemp protein, 1 tbsp. coconut oil

---

Blueberry Smoothie
1 banana, 2 cups of cold water, (or add 1 cup of ice and 1 ½ cups of water), 1/2 cup of blueberries, 1 tbsp ground flaxseed, 1 tbsp hemp protein, 1 tbsp agave nectar, 1 tbsp of hemp oil, 2 tsp. ground rooibos

---

Green Smoothie
6 leaves of romaine lettuce, 2 fresh or soaked dried dates, 2 cups of water, 1 cup of honeydew melon, 1 tbsp ground flaxseed, 1 tbsp hemp protein, ½ tbsp. grated fresh ginger

Other Healthy Drinks

Hot chocolate
Makes 1 serving

1 cup of almond milk, 1 packet stevia, 1 tablespoon pure cocoa powder

In saucepan, mix all ingredients. Stir over medium heat and serve.

Chai
1 cup almond milk, 1 packet of stevia, sprinkle cinnamon.

Condiments & Sauces

Quick guacamole

3 avocados
3 ripe jalapeno peppers
1 habanero pepper
3 tomatoes
1 bunch cilantro
1 ripe yellow lime

Mash ingredients together. Squeeze lime onto the mixture. If you keep the avocado pits in the mixture, this will help the guacamole to last longer.

Healthy Salsa

4 cups tomato
3 jalapeno peppers, seeds removed
3 garlic cloves, minced fine
1 onion

Juice from 2 limes
2 tsp Celtic sea salt
1 tbsp ground cumin
1 tbsp chili powder
1 cup sundried tomatoes, soaked in warm water
Cilantro leaves, whole
Basil leaves
½ of a red and yellow bell pepper, seeded

In a food processor, place the tomato, chopping into small pieces.

Place the jalapenos, garlic, onion, lime juice, salt, cumin, chili powder, and your choice of cilantro & basil into the food processor, chopping until very fine. Pour mixture into the bowl with the tomato. In the food processor, chop peppers until fine, putting them in the bowl with the tomato.

Place the sundried tomato into the food processor and process until smooth like tomato paste. Next mix this paste with the salsa in the bowl.

Original Hummus

2 zucchinis, peeled and chopped
1 cup raw tahini
½ cup fresh lime or lemon juice
½ cup cold pressed olive oil
¼ cup chopped olives (optional)
4 cloves garlic, minced
2 tsp celtic sea salt
½ tbsp ground cumin

In a high-speed blender, combine all ingredients and blend until thick and smooth.

Finally, Healthy Ketchup

3 tomatoes
3 pieces sundried tomatoes
5 dates (or 1/2 tsp stevia and 4 more sundried tomatoes)
1 squeeze of lemon juice
1/2 cup pure water

Put all ingredients in a blender. On the bottom of the blender, place the water, lemon juice and tomatoes. On top, add the sundried tomatoes and dates. Blend well. This will be easier if you soak the sundried tomatoes in water for a few hours.

Guacamole

3 avocados, chopped; juice of 2 limes; ¼ cup finely chopped red onion; 5 plum or vine-ripened tomatoes, chopped (or 1 cup grape tomatoes, sliced in half); ½ cup red or yellow peppers, diced; ½ bunch fresh cilantro, chopped; drizzle of olive oil; 1 packet of stevia; celtic sea salt to taste

Almond Milk (make your own almond milk)

1/2 cup almonds (soaked 12 hours)
1/2 cup pine nuts (soaked 6 hours)
1 cup spring or filtered water

Place soaked nuts in blender and pulverize. Gradually add one cup of water, while continuing to blend on high. Strain through a fine strainer or cheesecloth. Will keep for three to four days. You will love this on hot grains, such as quinoa, buckwheat groats, millet, or amaranth.

CHAPTER EIGHT
Exercise For Life

We have all heard it many times over. Exercise offers many health benefits – better sleep, reduced stress, less depression, higher self-esteem, improved strength and muscle tone and of course, weight loss. Regular exercise is one of the most important things you can do to improve your health and many of us do not realize how important exercise is until something bad happens to us. Your exercise life has to become a number one priority over everything else in your life.

Why circuit training is so important

Circuit training is an excellent way to simultaneously improve mobility, strength, stamina and lose weight. It provides excellent all round fitness, helps tone the body, builds your strength and is known to be one of the best ways to get maximum results in the shortest period of time. Circuit training places a unique type of stress on the body, compared to conventional weight training and aerobics. The fast pace and constant change shocks the body to create better results. I, myself, have tried just about every type of exercise routine and hands down, circuit training is one of the best to condition your entire body and mind.

Higher intensity exercise or lower intensity exercise?

When you work at a higher tempo your body uses less fat-fueled energy and it burns more carbohydrate-fueled energy. Many people get this wrong and say if you workout at a higher intensity, you will stop burning fat and only burn carbs. When you work out at a lower intensity you burn fewer calories. When you work at a higher intensity you burn more calories.

The real reason why you are exercising

To build lean muscle, strengthen your heart, reduce stress, burn fat, decrease your waist size, fight off disease, and the most important, to create healthy cells. Remember you're only as healthy as your cells are.

How to be happy

To release the pleasure centers in the brain, we must exercise to release the endorphins which in return will give you a sense of happiness and control, and in return, this will help you to eat less. It will also help you decrease depression and give you a more positive outlook on life.

Visualize

Visualization is probably one of the most underutilized success tools that you possess. Used correctly, visualization can take you to the next level in your weight and your life's goals.

1. Visualization is like a key to the subconscious mind. It activates the creative powers.

2. Visualization focuses your brain by programming its reticular activating system (RAS) to notice available resources that were always there but were previously unnoticed.

3. Visualization sends out the energy forces you need to attract the people, resources, and opportunities you need to achieve your goals.

Harvard University researchers found that students who visualized in advance performed tasks with nearly 100% accuracy, whereas students, who didn't visualize, achieved only 55% accuracy.

Your creative subconscious doesn't think in words; it can only think in pictures. When you give your brain specific, colorful, and vividly compelling pictures to manifest, it will seek out and capture all the information necessary to bring that picture into reality for you. If you give your mind an overweight problem, it will come up with a get-fit solution. If you give your mind a broke problem, it will come up with a make money solution. By contrast, if you are constantly feeding it negative, fearful and anxious pictures, it will give you exactly that.

Most people are visualizing what they don't want so that's exactly what they get. When your visualizing yourself as being overweight that's exactly what you get – you will be overweight. Start visualizing the weight you want to be at. You're confident, healthy and feeling great about yourself. That's exactly what you will get. It's the law of attraction.

Making Visualization work

Decide what you want, visualize it, go into the feeling of having it. Make the images as clear and as bright as possible. If your objective is to be at your ideal healthy weight, then close your eyes and see yourself being the exact person you would like to be.

Circuit one starts with a 30-second cardio warm up of jumping jacks, hand-to-knee taps or skipping.

Mental Repetition

Two minutes of mental repetition. Have the picture of the body you want in front of you. Look at the picture and then close your eyes for two minutes and visualize yourself having that body. How does it feel? What is your energy level? What do people say to you? How do you feel about yourself? See yourself walking around with that new amazing body.

Keep the picture in front of you during your workout.

Play fast tempo, uplifting, and motivational music while you're working out.

Circuit training is an excellent way to simultaneously improve mobility, strength, and stamina. The circuit training workout is composed of five different circuits, each having strength/cardio exercises that are completed one right after the other, with no rest in between. Perform one set of an exercise for a specific number of repetitions (or period of time) and then move on to the next exercise. When you have finished one set of each exercise in a circuit, you start back at the beginning of the circuit and repeat the exercises until you have completed the circuit three times.

For example, circuit one might include three sets each of squats, shoulder presses, and basic crunches. You should complete one set (consisting of 10 reps) of squats, followed by one set of shoulder presses and then one set of basic crunches, and then do a second set of squats, shoulder presses, and basic crunches, and then do the third and last set of the three exercises. Circuits must not consist of three sets of squats in a row, followed by three sets of shoulder presses and three sets of basic crunches.

There are no breaks in between the exercises of a single circuit; however, once you have fully completed a circuit, you can have a one-minute rest. The workouts contain cardio intervals (one minute of jumping jacks, one minute of hand-to-knee taps or skipping) to keep your heart rate up for a maximum calorie burn.

IMPORTANT: All cardio intervals are based on one minute

First, take 1 minute to sit and visualize the body you would like to have and the new person you would like to become. Start with a 30 second cardio warm up of jumping jacks, hand-to-knee taps or skipping.

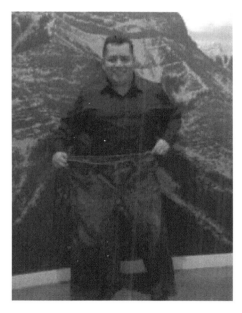

Fred has lost 43 pounds on the Think, Act, Love, Lose Weight program.

Week 1-3

Circuit routine (90 Days)

Perform exercise routine 4 days per week.

Rest 1 day.

Perform 30 minutes of cardio on your non-circuit training days. It could be a fast walk, or anything you enjoy.

CIRCUIT 1

REPEAT CIRCUIT
3 TIMES

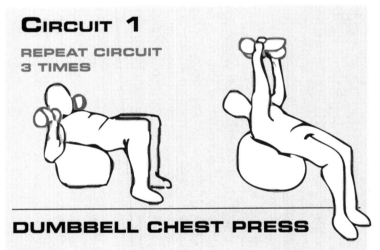

DUMBBELL CHEST PRESS

Step 1

Lie on your body ball with your feet firmly placed on the floor. Place dumbbells over your chest with your arms extended toward the ceiling, with both hands facing forward. You can use a workout bench.

Step 2

Slowly lower the weights to the side of your chest counting down to four. Raise the weights, again in an arc, and on the count of four, back to starting position.

Perform 10 reps.

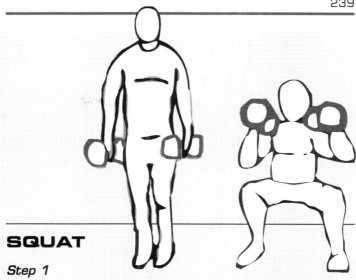

SQUAT

Step 1

Standing with your feet directly over your hips, keep your weight on your heels. Keep your shoulders directly over your hips. Hold a weight in each hand.

Step 2

Sit back down as if you were to sit down in a chair. Make sure you don't lean forward and keep your back straight. Lower yourself down on the count of four until your thighs are parallel with the floor. Straighten your legs, stand back up and repeat.

Step 3

To make it harder when you lower yourself down and you're coming back up, push the weights up over your head into a shoulder press and bring them back down on your way down.

Alternative: Leave your hands hanging to your sides with one in each hand, sit down in a chair and repeat.

Perform 10 reps.

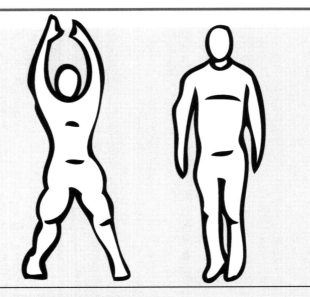

JUMPING JACKS
(hand- to- knee taps or skipping)

1 SET FOR 1 MINUTE

Step 1

Stand with your feet together, arms at sides, jump about hip width apart to shoulder

Step 2

Jump back and lower arms to starting position and re-peat

Tip: If you have bad knees, do hand taps. Touch your knee to each hand alternating for 1 minute. You can also substitute skipping for any of the cardio exercises for 1 minute.

1 minute rest between circuits.

Visualize the body you would like to have and the new person you are going to become.

Circuit 2

**REPEAT CIRCUIT
3 TIMES**

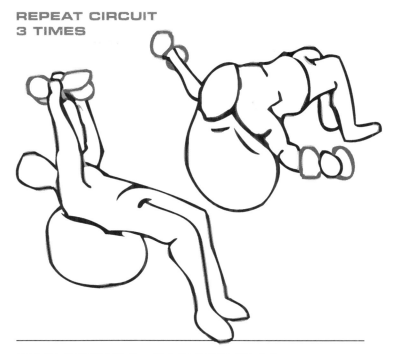

DUMBBELL CHEST FLY

Step 1

Lie on your body ball with your feet placed firmly on the floor. Place dumbbells over your chest with your arms extended toward the ceiling and both palms facing each other. You can use a workout bench.

Step 2

Slowly lower the weight to the side of your chest on the count of four. Raise the weight again in an arc, and back to starting position on the count of four.

Perform 10 reps.

FORWARD LUNGE

Step 1

Hold weights in each hand. Step forward with your left leg, leading with your heel.

Step 2

Make sure your left thigh is parallel to the floor and your right thigh is perpendicular to it. Do not lower yourself to 90 degrees. Place your legs in a 45- to 60-degree angle. Your right heel will slightly lift off the floor. Remember to push off the ball of your foot, step back into starting position and repeat with the opposite leg.

Perform 10 reps.

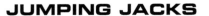

JUMPING JACKS

(hand- to- knee taps or skipping)

1 SET FOR 1 MINUTE

Step 1

Stand with your feet together, arms at sides, jump about hip width apart to shoulder

Step 2

Jump back and lower arms to starting position and repeat

1 minute rest between circuits.

Visualize the body you would like to have and the new person you are going to become.

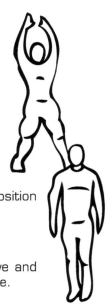

CIRCUIT 3

**REPEAT CIRCUIT
3 TIMES**

CHAIR DIP

Step 1

Stand with your back facing a bench or chair.
Place your hands on the edge of the bench or
chair. Most of your body weight should be on
your arms. It's important to keep your elbows
tucked into your sides.

Step 2

Lower yourself down on the count of
four until your arms are parallel and
push yourself back up and repeat.

Perform 10 reps.

PLANK

Step 1

Go into a push up position,
keeping your hands directly under your shoulders.
Your legs are straight behind you with your feet
together.

Step 2

Stay focused balancing on your palms and the balls
of your feet. Keep your abdominals tight.

Hold for one minute.

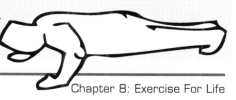

JUMPING JACKS

(hand- to- knee taps or skipping)

1 SET FOR 1 MINUTE

Step 1

Stand with your feet together, arms at sides, jump about hip width apart to shoulder

Step 2

Jump back and lower arms to starting position and repeat

1 minute rest between circuits. Visualize the body you would like to have and the new person you are going to become.

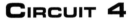

CIRCUIT 4

REPEAT CIRCUIT 3 TIMES

Shoulder press

Step 1

Using two dumbbells, with palms forward, grip and start with dumbbells at shoulder level. Press them overhead on the count of four.

Step 2

Lower the weights back to starting position on the count of four and repeat. Do not lock elbows at the top.

Perform 10 reps.

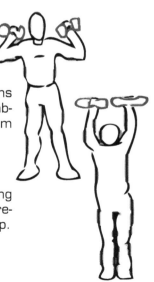

BASIC CRUNCH
WITH LEGS UP

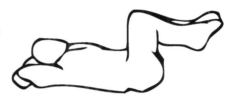

Step 1

Keep your eyes focused on the
ceiling and don't pull on your
neck. Curl up forward until your shoulders blades are lifted off the floor. Keep your legs up in the air.

Step 2

Lower back down to the
floor and repeat.

Perform 10 reps.

JUMPING JACKS
(hand- to- knee taps or skipping)
1 SET FOR 1 MINUTE

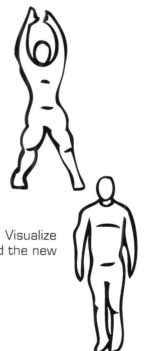

Step 1

Stand with your feet together,
arms at sides, jump about hip
width apart to shoulder

Step 2 .

Jump back and lower arms to
starting position and repeat

1 minute rest between circuits. Visualize
the body you would like to have and the new
person you are going to become.

Circuit 5

**REPEAT CIRCUIT
3 TIMES**

DUMBBELL TRICEP EXTENSION

Step 1

Keep your elbows close to your head and pointed straight up throughout the entire exercise. Raise the weights over your head.

Step 2

Lower back down to starting position and repeat.

Perform 10 reps.

BASIC CRUNCH

Step 1

Keep your eyes focused on the ceiling so you don't pull on your neck. Curl up forward until your shoulders blades are lifted off the floor on the count of four.

Step 2

Lower back down to the floor.

Perform 10 reps.

JUMPING JACKS
(hand- to- knee taps or skipping)
1 SET FOR 1 MINUTE

Step 1

Stand with your feet together, arms at sides, jump about hip width apart to shoulder

Step 2

Jump back and lower arms to starting position and repeat

Visualize: Take 5 minutes to cool down and visualize the person you want to become. Envision the body you're going to have and the feelings you have inside. Keeping moving at a slow pace.

Week 2-4

CIRCUIT 1

REPEAT CIRCUIT 3 TIMES

LATERAL SHOULDER RAISE

Step 1

Stand straight up with your feet shoulder width apart and your arms hanging to your sides. Hold a dumbbell in each hand with your palms turned toward your body. Keeping your arms straight, lift weights out to your sides until they are parallel to the ground.

Step 2

Lower your arms back to the starting position.

Perform 10 reps.

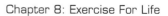

FORWARD LUNGE

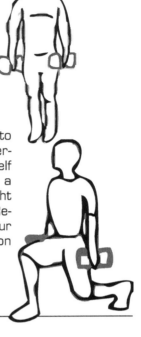

Step 1

Hold weights in each hand. Step forward with your left leg, leading with your heel.

Step 2

Make sure your left thigh is parallel to the floor and your right thigh is perpendicular to it. Do not lower yourself to 90 degrees. Have your legs in a 45- to 60-degree angle. Your right heel will slightly lift off the floor. Remember to push off the ball of your foot, step back into starting position and repeat with the opposite leg.

Perform 10 reps.

JUMPING JACKS

(hand- to- knee taps or skipping)

1 SET FOR 1 MINUTE
Step 1

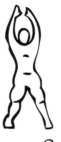

Stand with your feet together, arms at sides, jump about hip width apart to shoulder

Step 2

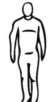

Jump back and lower arms to starting position and repeat

One minute rest between circuits. Visualize the body you would like to have and the new person you are going to become.

Think, Act, Love, Lose Weight

Circuit 2

REPEAT CIRCUIT 3 TIMES

SUPERMAN

Step 1

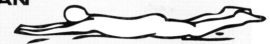

Lie on your stomach with your forehead on the floor and your arms straight out in front of you.

Step 2

Exhaling while lifting both arms and legs a couple inches off the floor.

Lower back down to the floor. Don't lift higher than a few inches off the floor.

Perform 10 reps.

PELVIC THRUST

Step 1

Lie on your back in front of the body ball, bench or platform with your knees bent and your heels on the body ball. Your legs should form a 90-degree angle with your knees directly above your hips, and your arms resting on the floor at your sides.

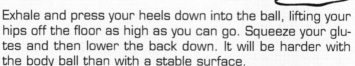

Step 2

Exhale and press your heels down into the ball, lifting your hips off the floor as high as you can go. Squeeze your glutes and then lower the back down. It will be harder with the body ball than with a stable surface.

Perform 10 reps.

JUMPING JACKS

(hand- to- knee taps or skipping)

1 SET FOR 1 MINUTE

Step 1

Stand with your feet together, arms at sides, jump about hip width apart to shoulder

Step 2

Jump back and lower arms to starting position and repeat

One minute rest between circuits. Visualize the body you would like to have and the new person you are going to become.

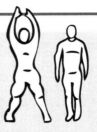

CIRCUIT 3

**REPEAT CIRCUIT
3 TIMES**

DUMBBELL BICEP CURL

Step 1

Place feet shoulder width apart. Hold a dumbbell in each hand facing toward the sides of your body. Keep your elbows locked firmly against your rib cage; curl both arms up towards your shoulders, rotating your wrist so your palm faces upward.

Step 2

Lower back down and repeat. Do not swing arms.

Perform 10 reps.

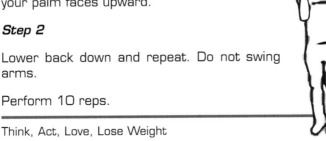

SQUAT

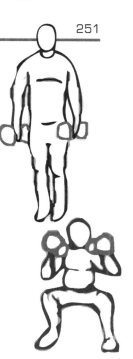

Step 1

Standing with your feet directly over your hips, keep your weight on your heels. Keep your shoulders directly over your hips. Hold weight in each hand.

Step 2

Sit back down as if you were to sit down in a chair. Make sure you don't lean forward and keep your back straight. Lower yourself down on the count of four until your thighs are parallel with the floor. Straighten your legs, stand back up and repeat.

Perform 10 reps.

JUMPING JACKS
(hand- to- knee taps or skipping)
1 SET FOR 1 MINUTE

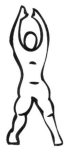

Step 1

Stand with your feet together, arms at sides, jump about hip width apart to shoulder

Step 2

Jump back and lower arms to starting position and repeat

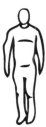

One minute rest between circuits. Visualize the body you would like to have and the new person you are going to become.

Circuit 4

REPEAT CIRCUIT
3 TIMES

FORWARD LUNGE

Step 1

Hold weights in each hand. Step forward with your left leg, leading with your heel.

Step 2

Make sure your left thigh is parallel to the floor and your right thigh is perpendicular to it. Do not lower yourself to 90 degrees. Have your legs in a 45- to 60-degree angle. Your right heel will slightly lift off the floor. Remember to push off the ball of your foot, step back into starting position and repeat with the opposite leg.

Perform 10 reps.

LATERAL SHOULDER RAISE

Step 1

Stand straight up with your feet shoulder width apart and your arms hanging to your sides. Hold a dumbbell in each hand with your palms turned toward your body. Keeping your arms straight, lift weights out to your sides until they are parallel to the ground.

Step 2

Lower your arms back to the starting position.

Perform 10 reps.

JUMPING JACKS

(hand- to- knee taps or skipping)

1 SET FOR 1 MINUTE

Step 1

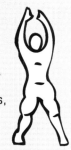

Stand with your feet together, arms at sides, jump about hip width apart to shoulder

Step 2

Jump back and lower arms to starting position and repeat

One minute rest between circuits. Visualize the body you would like to have and the new person you are going to become.

CIRCUIT 5

REPEAT CIRCUIT 3 TIMES

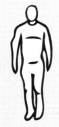

DUMBBELL CHEST FLY

Step 1

Lie on your body ball with your feet placed firmly on the floor. Place dumbbells over your chest with your arms extended toward the ceiling and both palms facing each other. You can use a workout bench.

Step 2

Slowly lower the weight to the side of your chest on the count of four. Raise the weight again in an arc, and back to starting position on the count of four.

Perform 10 reps.

BASIC CRUNCH

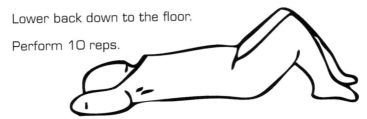

Step 1

Keep your eyes focused on the ceiling so you don't pull on your neck. Curl up forward until your shoulders blades are lifted off the floor on the count of four.

Step 2

Lower back down to the floor.

Perform 10 reps.

JUMPING JACKS

(hand- to- knee taps or skipping)

1 SET FOR 1 MINUTE

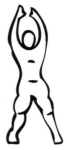

Step 1

Stand with your feet together, arms at sides, jump about hip width apart to shoulder

Step 2

Jump back and lower arms to starting position and repeat

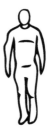

Visualize: Take 5 minutes to cool down and visualize the person you want to become. Envision the body you're going to have and the feelings you have inside. Keeping moving at a slow pace.

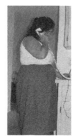 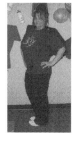

I am now a completely different woman. My confidence level has never been higher ever in my life. There are so many of Shane's teachings that I use in all areas of my life, not just for weight loss. I now have the ability to stay motivated every day. The quality of my life and relationships is at an all-time high. This was exactly the program I needed to keep the weight off forever. Finally I have stopped going from diet to diet.

- Tracy

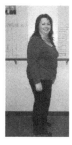 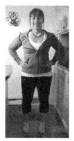

Shane teaches the mind-side of weight loss and fitness in a comprehensive, straight forward manner that makes success effortless! He provides the missing piece that most fitness professionals never address. Thanks Shane for guaranteeing my success!"

- Laura

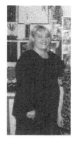 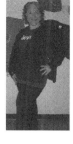

Shane has given me the missing link - the mind. It really has to be a 3 part strategy to take off the weight and keep it off. Thanks to Shane, I now have in my mind the strategies, anchors and the pictures to keep my weight off forever. I have been able to give myself permission to learn how to love myself. This book is a must for anybody who wants to lose weight and keep it forever.

- Penny

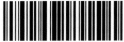
8116926R0